Essential Practices in Hospice and Palliative Medicine

Fifth Edition

Essential Practices in Hospice and Palliative Medicine
Fifth Edition

UNIPAC 4
NONPAIN SYMPTOM MANAGEMENT

Jennifer M. Kapo, MD
Yale University School of Medicine
New Haven, CT

Catherine Adams, MD PhD
The Community Hospice
St. Peter's Health Partners
Rensselaer, NY

Ryan M. Giddings-Connolly, MD
Mayo Clinic
Rochester, MN

Felicia Hui, MD
Stanford University School of Medicine
Stanford, CA

Andrew T. Putnam, MD
Yale University School of Medicine
New Haven, CT

Rebecca Sands, DO
University of Pittsburgh Medical Center
Pittsburgh, PA

Aleksander Shalshin, MD
Northwell Health
Syosset, NY

Reviewed by
James B. Ray, PharmD
The University of Iowa College of Pharmacy
Iowa City, IA

Edited by
Joseph W. Shega, MD
Vitas Healthcare
Miami, FL

Miguel A. Paniagua, MD FACP
University of Pennsylvania
Philadelphia, PA

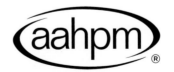

AMERICAN ACADEMY OF
HOSPICE AND PALLIATIVE MEDICINE

8735 W. Higgins Rd., Ste. 300
Chicago, IL 60631
aahpm.org | PalliativeDoctors.org

The information presented and opinions expressed herein are those of the editors and authors and do not necessarily represent the views of the American Academy of Hospice and Palliative Medicine. Any recommendations made by the editors and authors must be weighed against the healthcare provider's own clinical judgment, based on but not limited to such factors as the patient's condition, benefits versus risks of suggested treatment, and comparison with recommendations of pharmaceutical compendia and other medical and palliative care authorities.

Some discussions of pharmacological treatments in *Essential Practices in Hospice and Palliative Medicine* may describe off-label uses of drugs commonly used by hospice and palliative medicine providers. "Good medical practice and the best interests of the patient require that physicians use legally available drugs, biologics, and devices according to their best knowledge and judgment. If physicians use a product for an indication not in the approved labeling, they have the responsibility to be well informed about the product, to base its use on firm scientific rationale and on sound medical evidence, and to maintain records of the product's use and effects. Use of a marketed product in this manner *when the intent is the 'practice of medicine'* does not require the submission of an Investigational New Drug Application (IND), Investigational Device Exemption (IDE) or review by an Institutional Review Board (IRB). However, the institution at which the product will be used may, under its own authority, require IRB review or other institutional oversight" (US Food and Drug Administration, https://www.fda.gov/RegulatoryInformation/Guidances/ucm126486.htm. Updated January 25, 2016. Accessed May 17, 2017).

Published in the United States by the American Academy of Hospice and Palliative Medicine, 8735 W. Higgins Rd., Ste. 300, Chicago, IL 60631.

AAHPM Education Staff
Julie Bruno, Director, Education and Learning
Kemi Ani, Manager, Education and Learning
Angie Forbes, Manager, Education and Learning
Angie Tryfonopoulos, Coordinator, Education and
  Learning

AAHPM Editorial Staff
Jerrod Liveoak, Senior Editorial Manager
Bryan O'Donnell, Managing Editor
Andie Bernard, Assistant Editor
Tim Utesch, Graphic Designer
Jean Iversen, Copy Editor

ISBN 978-1-889296-24-1

Contents

Tables

Figures

Acknowledgments

AAHPM is deeply grateful to all who have participated in the development of this component of the Essential Practices in Hospice and Palliative Medicine self-study program. The expertise of the editors, contributors, and reviewers involved in the current and previous editions of the *Essentials* series has ensured the value of its content to our field.

AAHPM extends special thanks to the authors of previous editions of this volume: Rodney O. Tucker, MD MMM FAAHPM, Ashley C. Nichols, MD, Joel S. Policzer, MD FACP FAAHPM, Jason Sobel, MD, C. Porter Storey, Jr., MD FACP FAAHPM, and Carol F. Knight, EdM; the authors of the *UNIPAC 4* amplifire online learning module, Catherine Adams, MD PhD, Aleksander Shalshin, MD, and Patrick White, MD HMDC FACP FAAHPM; the pharmacist reviewer for this edition of the *Essentials* series, Jennifer Pruskowski, Pharm D; and the many professionals who volunteered their time and expertise to review the content and test this program in the field—Joe Rotella, MD MBA HMDC FAAHM, Joseph W. Shega, MD, Stacie Levine, MD, Marcin Chwistek, MD, John W. Finn, MD FAAHPM, Gerald H. Holman, MD FAAFP, Eli N. Perencevich, DO, and Julia L. Smith, MD.

Essential Practices in Hospice and Palliative Medicine was originally published in 1998 in six volumes as the UNIPAC self-study program. The first four editions of this series, which saw the addition of three new volumes, were created under the leadership of C. Porter Storey, Jr., MD FACP FAAHPM, who served as author and editor. AAHPM is proud to acknowledge Dr. Storey's commitment to and leadership of this expansive and critical resource. The Academy's gratitude for his innumerable contributions cannot be overstated.

Continuing Medical Education

Continuing medical education credits are available, and Maintenance of Certification credits may be available, to users who complete the *amplifire* online learning module that has been created for each volume of *Essential Practices in Hospice and Palliative Medicine*, available for purchase from aahpm.org.

Symptom Assessment Tools

Comprehensive assessment of patients is integral to providing holistic care and is made easier by the routine use of symptom assessment scales and other instruments. Because many of the symptoms important to overall quality of life (QOL) are subjective, thorough screenings and standards to document severity are needed for comparisons over time. Not only are symptoms such as pain, fatigue, nausea, depression, anxiety, poor appetite, and shortness of breath central to our care, but an understanding of how they affect each patient's life on a day-to-day basis is a priority as we strive to optimize QOL and discuss goal-oriented treatment. It also is important for palliative care clinicians to remember that symptoms often manifest in clusters; recognition of these clusters can help determine the best therapies in many situations in which one medication may treat more than one symptom.

Several symptom assessment scales have been validated in a variety of settings and patient populations and are available to quantify a patients' symptom experience. In a review of QOL tools for patients with cancer, proposed criteria for an ideal instrument include one that is simple to read and follow, quick and easy to complete and analyze, and based on a categorical or visual analog scale. The Edmonton Symptom Assessment Scale (ESAS) is a brief but relatively comprehensive measure of symptom burden for palliative care patients; multiple studies support its reliability and validity in cancer and noncancer populations. Additional measures that have been validated and incorporated into care include the Memorial Symptom Assessment Scale, the McGill Quality of Life Questionnaire, and the Functional Assessment Cancer Therapy.[1,2] Importantly, not all measures are relevant for all patient populations, and clinicians should carefully evaluate and select the most appropriate measures based upon the typical symptoms a population experiences. For example, the ESAS may identify and measure several relevant symptoms in dementia such as pain[3] and constipation but overlook other symptoms that impact QOL such as psychosis, agitation, and aggression.

For more information about these assessment tools, forms and instructions can be obtained through the National Palliative Care Research Center by visiting npcrc.org/content/25/Measurement-and-Evaluation-Tools.

Dyspnea

Clinical Situation

Dom and Nicola

Dom is a 46-year-old man with a 30-year history of heavy smoking. He was diag-nosed 12 months ago with adenocarcinoma of the right lung. He is an insurance agent who lives with his wife and two children in a new four-bedroom house in the suburbs. Dom has been struggling to go to work every day despite radiation treat-ments and has refused chemotherapy. He has been referred to your home-based hospice and palliative care program.

When the physician first visits, Dom is experiencing shortness of breath when he walks across the room. He is prescribed an albuterol inhaler, two puffs three times a day.

Further discussion reveals that Dom is using his albuterol inhaler approximately every hour during the day and is so tremulous and anxious that he gets little sleep at night. He is having moderate discomfort in his chest that is only slightly relieved by acetaminophen, but he refuses to take medications that might cause drowsiness because he wants to drive himself to work. An attempt at thoracentesis was made 2 weeks ago, but it was very painful and did not relieve Dom's dyspnea.

Dom is extremely angry with his employer, who has threatened to fire him because of his decreased work performance. Dom fears the likely cancellation of his health ben-efits and the loss of his home because, despite his career as an insurance agent, he has never purchased life insurance. He feels guilty about his lack of insurance and the probability that his family may have to leave their home as soon as his earnings stop. Dom's family is extremely stressed by his steady deterioration and increasing anger, which is often vented on Nicola and the children.

A physical examination reveals an angry, tremulous man who seems alert and clear-headed but appears older than his stated age. His blood pressure is 110/60 mm Hg, his pulse is 120, and his respirations are 30 breaths per minute. He has decreased breath sounds and scattered rhonchi in both lung fields, with absent breath sounds and dullness to percussion in the right lower lung field. His abdomen is soft with ten-derness in the epigastric area but no palpable mass. His extremities show some mus-cle wasting and clubbing of his fingertips but no cyanosis or edema.

As part of a multidimensional management approach, Dom's medications are altered with a decrease in the albuterol to two puffs three times day and beclomethasone inhaler added twice daily to help with bronchospasm. At the same time, the hospice nurse helps Dom set reasonable limits on his activities to avoid exhaustion (eg, use a wheelchair to conserve energy, allow family members to assist with family chores, allow someone to drive him to work). Finally, a social worker and chaplain become involved to address the family's financial problems and anguish about the future.

Dom's distress gradually improves as the above interventions are implemented. Several days later, lorazepam, 1 mg at bedtime, is added and Dom's sleep improves. His family begins to cope much better. With help from the social worker, Dom is able to negotiate a "when-needed" unpaid 6-month leave of absence with his employer, which allows him to retain his health insurance. However, 3 days later Dom begins to experience severe dyspnea. He is unable to return to work. Dom is not febrile or coughing up any sputum. The nurse listens to his chest and reports no major changes in his pulmonary examination.

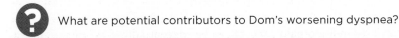 What are potential contributors to Dom's worsening dyspnea?

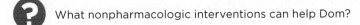 What nonpharmacologic interventions can help Dom?

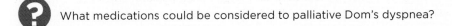 What medications could be considered to palliative Dom's dyspnea?

Definition and Prevalence

Dyspnea is a complex, uncomfortable sensation that includes air hunger, increased effort, and chest tightness. Sensory signals from the respiratory system are relayed to higher brain centers where they are processed and influenced by behavioral, cognitive, contextual, and environmental factors before the final sensation of breathlessness develops.[4] A 2011 neuroimaging study suggests that neural structures involved in pain and dyspnea might be shared; consequently, the neurophysiological and psychophysical approaches used to understand pain might be applied to dyspnea research.[5] Like pain, dyspnea is a subjective sensation that may be influenced by physical, psychological, social, and spiritual factors.

The complexity in pathophysiology leads to a wide variability in prevalence and intensity of dyspnea (**Table 1**).[6-12] Dyspnea has been reported to be the fourth most common reason for emergency department visits in the palliative care patient population. It is the reason for consultation in more than 10% of inpatient palliative care consultations.[13,14] Regardless of etiology, however, dyspnea tends to worsen as death approaches.[15]

Table 1. Prevalence of Dyspnea by Disease State[6-12]

Condition	Prevalence
Cancer (all types)	21%-70%
Cancer without cardiac or pulmonary pathology	24%
Cerebrovascular accident (stroke)	37%
Amyotrophic lateral sclerosis	50%
Chronic obstructive pulmonary disease	56%
Heart failure	61%-70%
HIV/AIDS	68%
Dementia	70%

Etiology and Pathophysiology

The etiology of dyspnea is complex, much like that of pain. In addition to the multiple potential pathophysiological etiologies, there are psychological, interpersonal, and existential domains that also contribute to the patient's experience and therefore shape the impact of the symptom for any patient. This multidomain concept can be conceptualized as "total dyspnea," similar to Cicely Saunders's concept of total pain, and has been described by Abernethy and colleagues.[16]

In broad physiological terms, patients may have large masses, pleural effusions, hypoxia or hypercapnia, bronchospasm, decreased cardiac output, anemia, or respiratory muscle weakness. These conditions cause afferent signals from chemoreceptors and mechanoreceptors in the airway, lungs, and chest wall, which are then sent to the respiratory center in the brain stem. This information is then transmitted to the cerebral cortex to integrate with cognitive and emotional input.

More specifically, the etiology of dyspnea may be divided into three general categories as described by Thomas and von Gunten[17]:

- work of breathing, caused by increased airway resistance or weakened muscles
- chemical causes, including hypercapnia (most important) and hypoxia
- neuromechanical dissociation (a mismatch between what the brain expects as respiration and the signals it receives).

Work of Breathing

Work of breathing is defined as increased respiratory effort induced by obstructive or restrictive pulmonary pathologies.[18] Conditions such as chronic obstructive pulmonary disease (COPD), thick bronchial secretions, and tracheobronchial malignant obstruction result in obstructive airway symptoms. Studies of patients with COPD suggest that the level of dyspnea is more significantly correlated to the 5-year survival rate than the traditional forced expiratory volume (FEV$_1$) measurement, and symptom management can improve the prognosis.[19,20]

Parenchymal and pleural pathologies such as pneumothorax, pneumonia, radiation pneumonitis, and pleural effusions lead to a restrictive picture. Intercostal muscle weakness from steroid myopathy, phrenic nerve damage, or other neurological conditions such as amyotrophic lateral sclerosis (ALS) can also induce dyspnea with a restrictive etiology, which in turn may be exacerbated by generalized fatigue or deconditioning.

Chemical Causes of Dyspnea

The chemical nature of breathing is better appreciated when remembering that oxygen is required to burn glucose during cellular metabolism, which in turn generates carbon dioxide and water. One may conceptualize oxygen as a nutrient and carbon dioxide as a waste product. When patients do not have enough nutrients, starvation occurs. When waste products build up, patients feel ill; for these reasons, hypoxia and hypercapnia are profound triggers for dyspnea.

Hypoxia may result from impaired diffusion of gases across the alveolar membrane by fluid or bacterial overload. On a more macroscopic level, hypoxia occurs when there is anemia or impaired cardiac pumping (eg, from myocardial ischemia, arrhythmia, valvular dysfunction, or pericardial effusion). In fact, several studies show that 50% of patients experiencing an acute myocardial infarction experience dyspnea.[21,22]

Carbon dioxide is a central player in acid-base homeostasis. In the respiratory process, it has been shown that hypercapnia increases dyspnea by stimulating the respiratory center in the medulla and peripheral mechanoreceptors. In paralyzed patients, increases in partial pressure of carbon dioxide induce the sensation of air hunger.[6] In situations inducing acidemia, such as sepsis, compensatory Kussmaul breathing occurs to blow off the acid load but also often leads to dyspnea.

Neuromechanical Dissociation

Neuromechanical dissociation is based on the theory of length-tension inappropriateness.[23] Normally there is an appropriate correlation between tension in the respiratory muscle and the resulting expansion of the lung parenchyma.[24] When the brain detects a discrepancy between these two components, the result may be the sensation of dyspnea.[25] For example, a pleural effusion may prevent a lung from expanding fully, even as a patient exerts an effort commensurate with the larger lung volume. Another patient may experience a tremendous amount of tension due to anxiety and take rapid, shallow breaths of which volumes are physiologically smaller than what would be expected for that tension.

Symptomatic Burden

The presence of dyspnea can have a profound effect on the QOL for both the patient and caregiver.[26] A review of more than 1,600 patients with severe COPD from the National

Emphysema Treatment Trial[27] showed a strong inverse relationship between dyspnea and health-related QOL, which was independent of FEV_1 measurements. An association between dyspnea and depression[28] has also been reported for patients with advanced cancer, including interference with general activity, mood, and enjoyment of life. In addition, the burden of such a profound symptom as dyspnea can easily extend beyond the patient and family to the healthcare staff and healthcare delivery system as a whole.

Assessment

Because of dyspnea's complex biopsychosocial etiology and subsequent manifestations, a standard assessment of this symptom becomes challenging. Given its subjective nature, the patient's self-report remains the gold standard for assessing its severity.[29] This is largely due to the lack of correlation between the sensation of dyspnea and objective measures such as respiratory rate, PCO_2, and PO_2. Therefore, some patients who are tachypneic indicate they are not dyspneic. Conversely, other patients who appear to be breathing comfortably even without noted hypoxia say they are very short of breath.[24]

Despite this, several validated tools exist for the assessment of dyspnea. The tools used for research purposes tend to focus on complex measurements of physiological parameters, and there has been an effort to develop assessment tools that focus more on the patient's experience of dyspnea. One such tool is the Cancer Dyspnea Scale, a 12-item multidimensional scale for patients with cancer that assesses effort, anxiety, and discomfort.[30] Additional assessment tools include the Modified Borg Scale and the Modified Research Council Scale, in which patients self-rate dyspnea severity on a 0 to 10 scale and self-rate how much activity is required to become breathless on a 0 to 4 scale; higher scores indicate worsening symptoms. However, there is not yet a single assessment tool that considers all aspects of this complex symptom that is easily incorporated into the clinical setting.[26] Thus, the best option is to assess dyspnea severity on a 0 to 10 numerical rating scale or the visual descriptor scale,[31] either independently or as part of a more complete review of symptoms, such as the ESAS.

For patients who are not able to self-report, an observational scale such as the Respiratory Distress Observation Scale can be used to assess eight items, including heart rate, respiratory rate, restlessness, paradoxical breathing, accessory muscle use, end expiratory grunt, nasal flaring, and fearful expression.[32] Each item is assigned a number from 0 to 2 with total scores of 0 to 16; higher scores indicate greater distress. The value of observational scales was bolstered by a recent prospective study[33] that demonstrated the subjective report of dyspnea by communicative patients in the intensive care unit (ICU) using a visual analog score strongly correlated with the Respiratory Distress Observational Scale.

When taking a patient's history and performing the physical examination, the clinician must attempt to clarify the primary cause or causes of dyspnea because each cause may necessitate a different intervention. If the history and physical examination are inconclusive of the etiology of dyspnea, additional tests may be indicated. Any proposed imaging study or procedure should take into account the patient's prognosis, goals of care, and the balance of the relative effort of procuring the test with the relative benefit of the associated intervention to alleviate the patient's symptoms. For example, a patient with cancer with a recurrent pleural effusion and an anticipated life expectancy of several months may be well palliated by thoracentesis and pleurodesis or an indwelling catheter. Of note, malignant pleural effusions tend to be better managed with an indwelling catheter because it avoids the initial hospital stay and leads to better symptom control[34] and fewer adverse events. In this case, a chest X-ray to start the evaluation is appropriate. However, this patient may decline further blood transfusions, which would make complete blood count testing unwarranted even if anemia may be contributing to dyspnea.

Management

The mnemonic presented in **Table 2** is a useful tool to help remember treatable abnormalities that trigger dyspnea. Depending on the severity and persistence of dyspnea, additional measures such as the use of opioids may be used for palliation (see **Figure 1**).

General Measures

Table 3 presents general measures for dyspnea treatment. Feeling dyspneic can be an acute emergency in the eyes of a patient. Although evaluating etiology and subsequent procedural and pharmacologic treatments is important, every member of the treating team (patient, family, and clinician) should have an action plan for dyspnea that includes immediate environmental changes that may help alleviate or lessen symptoms while waiting for further treatment.

All patients with dyspnea can benefit from proper positioning. When they are able, patients should be placed as vertically as possible to allow for optimal expansion of the rib cage by the intercostal and accessory muscles. Something as simple as changing positions can help relieve buildup of oral secretions and the presence of a "death rattle." In addition, if patients are not intuitively doing so, they should be instructed in the technique of pursed-lip breathing to increase expiratory airway pressure. There is evidence to support the benefits of oral opioids, neuromuscular electrical stimulation, chest-wall vibration, walking aids, and pursed-lip breathing in managing dyspnea for patients with advanced COPD.[36]

The simple act of placing a fan to blow cool air over the face is often valuable. A 2010 randomized study evaluated the efficacy of handheld fans to treat patients with refractory breathlessness caused by malignant and nonmalignant conditions; after only 5 minutes of having air blown directly on their face, patients showed a statistically significant decrease in breathlessness.[37] Although the mechanism of action is not fully understood, it may be that air flow stimulates the V_2 branch of the trigeminal nerve to decrease the perception of dyspnea.[38] Keeping the environment cool is also beneficial.

The presence of a companion at the bedside is an added intervention that often relieves isolation and anxiety. Patients will know they are not alone, and someone is present to call for help when needed.

Table 2. Specific Causes and Treatments for Dyspnea

B Bronchospasm.

Consider nebulized albuterol and ipratropium and/or an inhaled steroid such as inhaled beclomethasone twice daily. Systemic steroids can be useful in cases of superior vena cava obstruction or tumor mass effect in the lung.

R Rales.

If a patient is experiencing volume overload, reduce or stop intravenous fluids and artificial feeding. Diuretics may be helpful, particularly when cardiac output is low. If pneumonia appears likely, consider a trial of antibiotics based on the patient's goals of care, prognosis, and ability to take oral versus intravenous administration.

E Effusions.

Thoracentesis may be effective, and if the effusion recurs, pleurodesis or indwelling chest-tube drainage may be appropriate based on goals of care and an anticipated life expectancy of at least several weeks to months.

A Airway obstruction, aspiration.

Make sure that tracheostomy appliances are cleaned regularly. If aspiration of food is likely, puree solids and thicken liquids with cornstarch. Educate the family about how to position the patient during feeding. Suction the patient when appropriate.

T Thick secretions.

If the cough reflex is still strong, loosen thick secretions with nebulized saline and guaifenesin. If the cough is weak, treat thin secretions with atropine, 1% ophthalmic solution, 1-4 drops sublingually every 4 hours or as needed; 1-3 patches of topical scopolamine (1.5 mg/patch) behind the ear(s) every 3 days; or glycopyrrolate (lowest risk of delirium with use), 0.2-0.4 mg subcutaneous or intravenous bolus every 3 hours as needed.

H Hemoglobin low.

A blood transfusion may add energy and reduce dyspnea for a few weeks. As always, however, the clinician needs to discuss the clinical status and goals with the patient and family to help determine the potential benefits versus relative burden of the transfusion, especially taking into consideration the etiology (and speed of recurrence) of the anemia.

Continued on page 10

Table 2. Specific Causes and Treatments for Dyspnea *(continued)*

A Anxiety.

Sitting upright, using a bedside fan, listening to calming music, and practicing relaxation techniques can be effective, as can skillful counseling and the presence of a calming clinician. When chronic anxiety is believed to be a trigger for dyspnea, clonazepam or antidepressants may be helpful. Keeping this in mind, dyspnea is a potent trigger for anxiety and may best be treated with opioids first and then a benzodiazepine. If the opioid dosage is limited by drowsiness, reduce the benzodiazepine dosage and then attempt to increase the opioid dosage.

I Interpersonal issues.

Social and financial problems contribute to anxiety and dyspnea. Counseling and interaction with social workers and other members of the interdisciplinary team may bring relief. When family relationships exacerbate the problem, a few days spent in a peaceful, home-like hospice inpatient unit may help to relieve the patient's symptoms.

R Religious concerns.

Although faith or an experience of the transcendent can bring profound comfort, some beliefs, such as "God is punishing me" or "God will heal me if I have enough faith," can precipitate or exacerbate dyspnea. Take the time to listen with full attention and presence, encouraging the patient to explore ways to reconnect and relieve existential burden. Coordinate treatment with the patient's spiritual adviser, chaplain, counselor, other healthcare professionals, and family members.

Figure 1. Global Therapies for Dyspnea Management

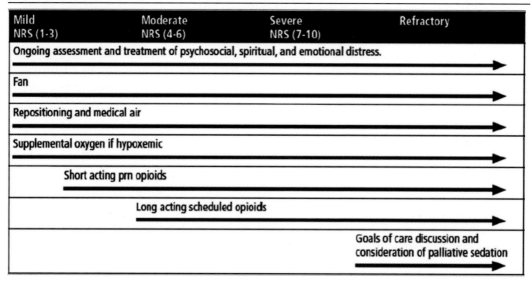

Table 3. Nonpharmacologic Measures to Treat Dyspnea

Reduce the need for exertion and arrange for readily available assistance with transfers, ambulation, activities of daily living, feeding, or any other activities known to trigger dyspnea.

Reposition the patient, usually to a more upright position or with the compromised lung down.

Improve air circulation:
- Provide a draft by using fans or opening windows.
- Adjust humidity with a humidifier or air conditioner.
- Avoid strong odors, fumes, and smoke.
- Increase flow of oxygen temporarily until symptoms improve.

Address anxiety and provide reassurance:
- Discuss the need for companionship and spiritual support because isolation and spiritual concerns can exacerbate symptoms.
- Discuss the meaning of symptoms and other patient or family concerns.
- Anticipate and rehearse with the patient and family their responses when symptoms worsen.
- Identify situational components (such as things that trigger dyspnea attacks).
- Teach relaxation interventions such as abdominal breathing or hypnosis.
- Consider rehabilitative strategies such as breathing training, relaxation, and adaptive strategies.[35]

Oxygen

Supplemental oxygen therapy is commonly used to palliate dyspnea. This is often because it is considered an expected therapy by patients and families despite any doubts clinicians may have regarding its efficacy.[39] The value of oxygen in patients with severe hypoxemia with dyspnea is not in question. Landmark studies[40,41] have demonstrated both survival and QOL benefits in hypoxemic patients with COPD. Studies have also shown that patients with COPD who are nonhypoxemic at rest but develop hypoxemia with activity achieve improved QOL and reduced dyspnea with the use of oxygen.[42] For patients who are nonhypoxemic with COPD, there is significant heterogeneity between studies, and there is no firm evidence to support the use of oxygen.

The use of oxygen in a more generalized palliative care population and, specifically, for patients with only mild hypoxemia or without hypoxemia is more controversial.[43] Despite this, prescribing palliative oxygen is a common practice, with more than 70% of physicians prescribing oxygen therapy for palliative care patients with refractory dyspnea for either palliation of symptoms or upon patient request.[44] An evaluation of the evidence base[45] for oxygen use in refractory breathlessness in advanced disease elucidated some important research questions that still need to be addressed. These include whether oxygen itself or the flow of cool air contributes more to the reduction of dyspnea and the effect on the dyspnea for those near the end of life.

A large, double-blinded, randomized controlled trial conducted by Abernethy and colleagues made some headway at answering these questions. More than 200 nonhypoxemic patients with refractory dyspnea due to a life-limiting illness received either oxygen or medical air (room air with ambient partial pressure of oxygen) via nasal cannulae for more than 15 hours per day for 7 days. Over the study period, both oxygen and medical air improved dyspnea ratings and QOL ratings, indicating that the main benefit may be from the sensation of moving air alone. In addition, this study reported that those patients with a higher baseline level of dyspnea received greater benefit than those with a lower baseline level of dyspnea and that the most benefit occurred in the first 48 to 72 hours.

A double-blind, n-of-1 trial[46] looked at the routine use of oxygen in patients nearing death. In this study, 100 patients who were either enrolled in hospice or were being evaluated by an inpatient palliative care service were observed for respiratory distress as medical air, oxygen, and no-flow were randomly alternated every 10 minutes via nasal cannulae over the period of an hour. The range of hypoxemia varied greatly in the study; however, there was no significant change in the display of respiratory distress for any of the patients.

In light of this evidence, the British Thoracic Society recently revised their guidelines[47] for the use of oxygen therapy, stating that patients with cancer or end-stage cardiorespiratory disease who are nonhypoxemic should be assessed for opioid or fan therapy before palliative oxygen therapy. They suggest that palliative oxygen therapy should only be considered on an individual basis when symptoms are refractory to all other treatments.

Similarly, The American Thoracic Society[48] recommends the use of supplemental oxygen for patients receiving palliative care in the context of pulmonary rehabilitation for those with moderate to severe dyspnea but confirms that there is no firm evidence for its use in the absence of hypoxemia.

Opioids

Opioids are considered first-line pharmacologic agents for managing nonspecific dyspnea for patients with advanced disease.[49] Although their mechanisms for relieving dyspnea are not well understood, they may decrease the chemoreceptor response to hypercapnia, increase peripheral vasodilatation with a decrease in cardiac preload, or decrease anxiety with the result of altering the perception of dyspnea.[50-52] Opioids also have been shown to increase exercise tolerance for patients with COPD,[53] improve dyspnea for patients with chronic congestive heart failure (CHF),[54] and mitigate dyspnea for patients with terminal cancer.[55] A *Cochrane* meta-analysis found that opioids have a small but statistically significant positive effect on breathlessness, although the quality of the studies needs improvement.[56] They may alter the perception of dyspnea at different levels of the afferent pathways.[57] For COPD, there is evidence that opioids inhibit the respiratory center's sensitivity to hypercapnia.[17]

A wide variety of opioids has been demonstrated to mitigate dyspnea. Conventional wisdom holds that morphine is a better agent than other opioids for dyspnea relief, and the literature does not support or refute this; however, no studies demonstrate one opioid as having clear benefits over others. Morphine is the most studied opioid for the relief of dyspnea,[58] which may account for its presumed superiority. Although there is no consensus regarding opioid dosages, **Table 4** lists the American Thoracic Society's End-of-Life Task Force[48] recommendations for initiating opioids for adult palliative care patients with moderate to severe dyspnea.

Keeping these general guidelines in mind, the clinician needs to determine, with the assistance of the caregiver and interdisciplinary team, the appropriate dosage and interval to achieve adequate dyspnea relief. The time to peak plasma concentration for the oral opioid formulations is generally 1 hour, so if the dosage is not sufficient, it may be safely titrated upward by 25% to 50% every 2 hours until dyspnea relief is achieved. If the dosage is sufficient but the interval between doses is too long, more frequent dosing is warranted, even on an hourly basis. The goal of such careful titration is to systematically find the lowest effective dose. To treat dyspnea for opioid-tolerant patients, the patient's existing opioid regimen is titrated to efficacy. If the opioid is taken on an as-needed basis and the dosage is sufficient to provide relief, schedule the medication every 4 hours in addition to adding a rescue dose every 3 to 4 hours as needed. If the patient is taking hydrocodone or codeine and has severe dyspnea, consider rotating the opioid to a more potent agent such as morphine or hydromorphone. Opioid rotation is also helpful when titration is limited by adverse side effects such as confusion or nausea. Intermittent subcutaneous (SC) morphine infusions have also been shown to be effective for relief of dyspnea.[59] This may be particularly useful when patients have difficulty swallowing medications or need more rapid symptom relief than can be achieved by oral administration, but intravenous access is not available.

In cases of chronic dyspnea or refractory symptoms, patients may need scheduled doses of opioids to keep their dyspnea under consistent control. In this situation, changing to a long-acting opioid formulation has been shown to be effective. A randomized, blinded, placebo-controlled trial revealed efficacy of long-acting morphine, 20 mg by mouth daily, showing decreased subjective breathlessness and better sleep.[60] A dose-finding study of a once-daily, slow-release morphine product for dyspnea suggested that 10 mg daily was generally effective and well tolerated.[61]

The nebulization of opioids is intriguing, given the theory that inhaled opioids may act directly on airway receptors resulting in lower systemic absorption and therefore fewer adverse effects. In addition, their onset of action is thought to be significantly shorter than traditional oral opioids, which is particularly useful when used for episodic periods of dyspnea. Although some early studies showed improvement in the perception of dyspnea with nebulized fentanyl,[55] subsequent review of the literature has not resulted in any firm evidence that nebulized or intranasal opioids are effective.[62,63] A *Cochrane* review[56] on the use of opioids

Table 4. Starting Opioid Dosages for Moderate to Severe Dyspnea for Adults Receiving Palliative Care

Agent	IV	Oral
Oxycodone	N/A	5-10 mg every 3-4 hours
Morphine	2-10 mg every 3-4 hours	5-10 mg every 3-4 hours
Hydromorphone	0.3-1.5 mg every 3-4 hours	2-4 mg every 3-4 hours
Fentanyl	50-100 mcg every 0.5-1 hour	N/A

IV, intravenous; N/A, not available

for refractory breathlessness in advanced illness found no evidence for the use of nebulized opioids. Similarly a consensus statement from the American College of Chest Physicians agrees that although a trial of nebulized opiates can be considered, there is no evidence to support relief of breathlessness.[49]

The issue of opioid safety has long been a topic of discussion, especially when respiratory parameters are of importance. The historic barrier to the use of opioids for the relief of dyspnea has been the concern for respiratory depression. Although respiratory depression is possible, in the setting of proper management this fear is largely unfounded. Clemens and colleagues[64,65] evaluated changes in respiratory parameters, including oxygen saturation, arterial pressure of carbon dioxide, respiratory rate, and pulse during titration of morphine or hydromorphone for the relief of dyspnea. A decrease in respiratory rate was observed without changes in the other parameters, and the patients reported a significant improvement in their dyspnea. A 2014 article[66] confirmed that opioids used for symptomatic relief of dyspnea do not significantly impact respiratory function. It is important to remember that opioids should be used for respiratory distress (subjectively reported dyspnea or common signs of distress such as nasal flaring, grunting, and retractions), not for isolated tachypnea. Respiratory depression follows sedation; consequently, the clinician needs to observe the patient's mental status. Significant depression of breathing is unlikely to occur when the patient is alert or easily aroused; in this situation naloxone is not appropriate. When the patient has been on a stable opioid regimen for more than several days and subsequently develops mental status changes, the clinician must consider other underlying culprits because the patient likely has already developed a tolerance to the sedative effects of opioids. The workup at this point is similar to that for acute delirium, with the possibility of infectious causes or metabolic derangements being high on the differential diagnosis because these may amplify the neurocognitive effects of opioids. In the case of either significant respiratory depression or sedation, the concept of double effect should be considered. In other words, the clinician must take into account the patient's treatment preferences and prognosis and discuss with the surrogate decision makers ways in which to balance the need for symptom management and the desire to restore alertness or potentially prolong life.

Despite this evidence, there remain many concerns about the potential for opioids to induce respiratory depression. Providers may consider using naloxone when a patient's respiratory rate drops. Palliative medicine clinicians need to educate patients, families, and healthcare providers about the effects of opioids on respiration and how to tailor a plan of action when respiratory depression is present. Naloxone completely blocks opioid receptors. Therefore, it needs to be used judiciously so as to not unnecessarily reverse the desired effects of pain and dyspnea relief. Ultimately the use of naloxone should be limited to rare instances of accidental opioid overdose or inadvertent overmedication. It should be administered in a way that minimizes the risk of completely reversing the effects of opioids. One ampule of naloxone (0.4 mg) should be diluted in 10 mL of normal saline and then given in 1 mL aliquot portions (0.04 mg) intravenously every 5 minutes until partial reversal occurs.[67] The patient requires close observation, with the expectation that further aliquot portions may be needed because naloxone has a shorter half-life than most opioids.[68] Long-acting opioids are commonly used by opioid-tolerant patients with chronic, life-threatening illness; in cases of mental status changes, however, it may be more sensible to hold further dosages and to wait for opioid washout rather than to repeatedly administer naloxone.

When a patient is nearing death, changes in the respiratory pattern may occur. Specifically the patient's breathing may become irregular with periods of apnea or full Cheyne-Stokes respiration. Respiration may also become noisy with end-expiratory moaning. These changes in respiration usually indicate that the patient is undergoing the normal dying process and does not necessarily indicate respiratory distress. Opioid titration is often not necessary unless there are other signs of pain or suffering. It is important to educate those at the bedside, both caregivers and family members, regarding these changes and provide reassurance and emotional support.

Anxiolytics

Patients with severe dyspnea often experience a vicious cycle in which the dyspnea induces anxiety, which in turn amplifies dyspnea. Anxiolytics have been specifically studied for the relief of dyspnea; however, most studies have failed to show a beneficial effect in patients with advanced cancer and COPD.[69,70] Navigante and colleagues compared the use of oral midazolam with oral morphine in the outpatient setting and found that midazolam was more effective after 5 days, although the duration of this study was short, making any generalizations a challenge.[71] A 2016 prospective study on the safety of benzodiazepines and opioids showed that benzodiazepines alone had a dose-response trend associated with mortality, however low-dose opioids used concurrently with benzodiazepines did not.[72] The US Food and Drug Administration (FDA) released a drug safety statement highlighting serious safety concerns about prescribing a combination of opioids and benzodiazepines for patients who are not at the end of life because of the increased risk of respiratory depression.[73] Notably, a *Cochrane Database* systematic review concluded that there is "no evidence for or against benzodiazepines for the relief of breathlessness in people with advanced cancer and COPD."[70] Most experts agree that benzodiazepines should be reserved as second- or third-line treatment used for breakthrough or refractory dyspnea compounded by anxiety symptoms, when other interventions have failed, or when undue side effects limit titration of opioids to efficacy.[71]

Alprazolam may be too short acting for this indication, but clonazepam can produce 8 to 12 hours of coverage, which is useful in cases of chronic dyspnea. A recommended starting regimen is clonazepam, 0.25 mg orally every 12 hours. Lorazepam offers some of both benefits, providing more rapid onset than clonazepam but lasting for 4 to 6 hours. Moreover, lorazepam is available in an oral concentrate that can be administered sublingually when oral intake is difficult. The combination of an opioid and lorazepam has been shown to relieve dyspnea without significant respiratory depression;[74] however, sedation can occur. When a parenteral infusion is needed to deliver the opioid, adding midazolam to the infusion can be helpful for severe, refractory dyspnea.[75] Given the potential risks of combined opioid and benzodiazepine administration discussed above, many specialists recommend prescribing naloxone and educating patients on their use to prevent inadvertent overdose, especially for patients cared for in ambulatory settings who may not be at the end of life.[43,73]

Management of Congestion and Secretions

Congestion and pulmonary edema can be significant causes of dyspnea, and patients with end-stage CHF may experience a "revolving door" of admissions for parenteral diuresis near the end of life. Anecdotal success of intermittent subcutaneous furosemide therapy for at-home diuresis prompted a 2011 study evaluating the efficacy of continuous subcutaneous furosemide infusions to prevent hospital readmissions and control symptoms for patients who were dying. Data revealed that 93% of the 28 patients were successful in avoiding rehospitalization, with 70% success in weight loss (consistent with effective diuresis).[76] Of the additional 15 patients actively dying, symptoms were controlled in 100%.[76] Although initial success using subcutaneous furosemide is encouraging, continued research in these patient populations can lead to significant improvement in outcomes. For more detailed information regarding treatment of pulmonary edema associated with heart failure, see *UNIPAC 8*.

In addition to pulmonary edema leading to congestion and dyspnea, upper airway secretions (also referred to as the "death rattle") can occur. Although these secretions may be perceived to be a troubling symptom at the end of life, most research shows a lack of correlation between the presence of upper airway secretions and respiratory distress. In addition, there is no evidence to support that treatments of these secretions are effective in reducing the intensity or presence of the death rattle.[77] Nevertheless, multiple medications for cough and those intended to thicken or thin secretions anecdotally have been helpful.

Anticholinergics are most often used because their side effect profile can be relied upon to dry up secretions and congestion; different formulations of these medications can be chosen based on a patient's clinical scenario. Glycopyrrolate is available in oral and intravenous forms but also can be given subcutaneously if needed; its quick onset of action, as well as its resistance to crossing the blood-brain barrier and increasing somnolence, make it ideal in the palliative setting. Scopolamine also is available as a patch, allowing for easy administration in the home setting. Similarly atropine drops can be given buccally to unresponsive patients to help with oral secretions. For information about dosing of these medications, refer to Table 2. Although these medications can be helpful, especially if secretions are distressing to patients and families, remember that anticholinergics can contribute to other symptoms such as dry mouth, constipation, urinary retention, and delirium (except for glycopyrrolate) and should be carefully monitored. These medications do not eliminate material already in the airways, so aspiration still may occur. In addition, drying up pulmonary secretions may place the patient at risk for inspissation of secretions and mucous plugging.[78] In addition to the above interventions, it is important to consider discontinuing therapies that may be contributing to both pulmonary edema and upper airway secretions, such as intravenous fluids and enteral or parenteral nutrition.

A 2008 *Cochrane* review of this subject concluded

> There is currently no evidence to show that any intervention, be it pharmacological or nonpharmacological, is superior to placebo in the treatment of death rattle. We acknowledge that in the face of heightened emotions when death is imminent, it is difficult for staff not to intervene. It is therefore likely that the current therapeutic options will continue to be used. However, patients need to be closely monitored for lack of therapeutic benefit and adverse effects while relatives need time, explanation, and reassurance to relieve their fears and concerns. There is a need for more well-designed multi-centre studies with objective outcome measures and the ability to recruit sufficient numbers.[79]

Complementary and Alternative Medicine Interventions

Some patients may wish to pursue complementary modalities such as acupuncture to better alleviate their dyspnea. Complementary and alternative medicine modalities have been primary modalities in other societies and cultures and have garnered tremendous interest by the American public. Modalities relevant to dyspnea management include acupuncture, acupressure, massage, and meditative practices,[80] yet related studies remain small in sample size and few in number.

Several studies explore the use of acupuncture in comparison to sham-needle use for patients with cancer and COPD; many of these studies reveal equivocal increased benefit for acupuncture and demonstrate the power of the placebo effect.[81-83] In 2012, however, a study conducted in Japan compared acupuncture with sham needling in patients with dyspnea on exertion from underlying COPD who were also receiving standard medication.[84] This randomized, controlled trial showed significant improvement in the 6-minute walk test and QOL for the patients receiving acupuncture after 12 weeks.

Noninvasive Ventilatory Support

Noninvasive ventilatory support is defined as ventilatory support without the use of an endotracheal device. The least invasive of these techniques is high-flow nasal cannula, which combines oxygen with pressurized air and warm humidification to allow up to 40 L per minute of oxygen flow. High-flow nasal cannula may be better tolerated than other forms of noninvasive positive-pressure ventilation (NPPV), allowing patients to retain the ability to eat, clear secretions, and communicate.[85] If, however, a patient is not improving and wishes to go home, the ability of the home hospice or home care service to provide oxygen flow of 30 L to 40 L per minute should be considered before instituting this therapy because weaning a patient in respiratory distress may be difficult. More studies are needed regarding the ways in which this therapy might be used in settings outside of acute inpatient facilities.

Alternative modalities to provide ventilatory support include different types of NPPV. These include continuous positive airway pressure (CPAP), which provides supplemental pressure on inspiration, and bilevel positive airway pressure (BiPAP), which provides supplemental pressure on both inspiration and expiration. Both devices use a tight mask to deliver pressure in the range of 5 cm to 14 cm water. In recent years these methods have been used more frequently for patients with chronic respiratory failure, increasing their ability to speak, swallow, and eat even with these devices in place and decreasing the risks associated with endotracheal intubation such as airway and lung injury and nosocomial pneumonias.[86,87]

CPAP and BiPAP are best used for cognitively intact patients who are hemodynamically stable and not agitated when wearing the required tight-fitting mask. Observational studies that have looked at the use of NPPV in the setting of hypercapnic respiratory failure show similar success among comatose and noncomatose patients, suggesting that at least a trial of its use may be justified based on family goals to determine whether a component of hyperbaric encephalopathy may be reversible.[88]

NPPV has been shown to be beneficial for a number of different patient populations. For instance, a small subset of patients with COPD may benefit from supplemental pressure at night. In addition, patients with neurodegenerative disorders may benefit from these devices as their respiratory muscles weaken.[89,90] Similarly, in a large study of more than 1,000 patients with acute cardiogenic pulmonary edema, NPPV was effective in resolving patients' dyspnea but was not associated with significant improvement in patient mortality.[91]

The use of noninvasive ventilatory support for cancer patients or those nearing the end of life is more controversial. A feasibility trial showed the use of both high-flow oxygen and BiPAP to be safe and effective for hospitalized patients with refractory dyspnea and advanced cancer[92]; however, additional larger scale studies are needed to clarify the benefit in this patient population. This is because the ratio of burden to benefit in these cases is very unclear.

In a study reported in the *Journal of Palliative Medicine* in 2014, Quill proposed that NPPV may be beneficial for dying patients with preexisting do not attempt resuscitation directives if used as a bridge while disease-directed therapy or palliative therapies are given the chance to work.[93] In these cases, NPPV is used as a time-limited trial, and clear endpoints should be established before initiating therapy. If, at any time, the intervention becomes overly burdensome or uncomfortable, it should be discontinued because it may interfere with the primary goal of comfort.[94]

Even though CPAP and BiPAP do not involve an invasive endotracheal tube, they may be bothersome for patients. The straps or masks themselves may cause discomfort or induce claustrophobia, and patients may object to the sensation of supplemental airway pressure or the noisy airflow. Among otherwise healthy patients prescribed CPAP for sleep apnea, 85% do not continue with the treatment unless they receive cognitive behavioral therapy to help them tolerate it.[95]

Over the course of a patient's illness, clinicians need to continually reassess the relative merits and disadvantages of ventilatory support with the patient, surrogate decision maker or caregiver, and interdisciplinary team. What is the purpose of this intervention at this point in time? Is it likely or even possible that the patient may enjoy weeks of life on such therapy? Is it more desirable to be as alert and interactive as possible and acknowledge that these modalities will prolong the dying process? Or is it more desirable for the patient to stop any intervention that prolongs the dying process or causes discomfort and refocus on methods that only promote relief of dyspnea? The clinician can help the patient and family reassess their goals and potentially explore the time at which the patient may consider stopping this intervention. It is also important to clearly document the conversations that lead to these decisions to best communicate with other members of the healthcare team.[96]

Refractory Dyspnea

When a clinician encounters a patient who is experiencing refractory and severe dyspnea that is not amenable to the aforementioned modalities, he may then consider the desirability and appropriateness of proportional palliative sedation, described as the use of the minimum amount of sedation necessary to relieve refractory physical symptoms at the end of life.[97] Two critical features of therapeutic sedation clearly distinguish it from euthanasia: (a) the goal is to relieve dyspnea (or other uncontrolled symptom burden), not to hasten death, and (b) a protocol is in place to titrate the medication downward at predetermined intervals to reassess whether the underlying symptom is still apparent. However, breakthrough dyspnea may necessitate titrating medications upward, thus decreasing overall alertness and, unfortunately, interaction with loved ones.

In this situation, the clinician must have a frank and thoughtful discussion with the patient, when possible, or decision makers to reassess goals of care, ensure that therapeutic sedation is consistent with these goals, and explain the specific method used to achieve this goal and how this intervention will be reassessed over time to ensure it is still needed. The section on palliative sedation in *UNIPAC 6* further describes a suggested process for discussing therapeutic sedation with patients or decision makers, obtaining informed consent, clarifying which medications to use, and reassessing ongoing use of such medication.

Compassionate Ventilator Withdrawal

Patients with complex needs at the end of life often require the help of physicians with many skills. There is increasing discussion of the responsibilities of hospice and palliative medicine and pulmonary and critical care physicians in providing end-of-life care to patients and their families.[98] Tasks and issues include prognostication and decision making about goals of care, challenges and approaches to communicating with patients and their families, the role of interdisciplinary collaboration, principles and practices of withholding and withdrawing life-sustaining measures, and cultural competence in end-of-life care.[99]

An ethics committee consultation can be helpful in complex cases.[100] Excellent information is available about managing cases of dying patients in the ICU; resources include discussions of the practical, legal, and ethical aspects of end-of-life ventilator withdrawal.[101-103] As more research is conducted in this area, and physicians with different skill sets collaborate, patient care at the end of life in the ICU is likely to improve.

There is no standardized method or protocol for removing mechanical ventilation. Both removal of the endotracheal tube (extubation) and gradual reduction of oxygen concentration and ventilatory support (weaning) have been used. In either case, patients should be adequately medicated to prevent discomfort or distress.[48,104] A review article by Rubenfeld outlines some useful principles for ventilator withdrawal.[105]

Dysphagia

Clinical Situation

Jamen

Jamen is a 92-year-old man with a history of Parkinson's disease and dementia that has been progressing for several years. He is transferred from a long-term-care facility to an area hospital with symptoms of aspiration pneumonia and respiratory distress. After initial resuscitation, antibiotics, and supportive clinical therapy, Jamen's condition improves.

A speech and swallow assessment is performed 24 hours after initial presentation, which demonstrates oropharyngeal dysphagia with decreased mastication and pooling of secretions. The results are reported to Jamen's family, who requests a second opinion for guidance on how to proceed. A palliative care physician is consulted for assessment of goals of care, feeding options, and overall prognosis.

On exam Jamen appears weak and frail, unable to answer questions, and responsive to tactile and painful stimulation. Poor dentition, weakness of musculature, and dysarthria are noted. Jamen is unable to cough up secretions that are pooling in the back of this throat and is unable to perform independent activities of daily living or basic activities of daily living. Jamen's family agrees to a trial of oral-assisted feeding and aspiration precautions. They are educated on elevating the head of Jamen's bed, assisted feeding, and provision of small frequent meals and liquid supplements. Elimination of dietary restrictions is also recommended. Initially Jamen seems to be taking small amounts of food by assisted oral feeding and maintaining a decent caloric intake. However, over the course of the next 24 to 48 hours, he has refused offers of assisted feeding, at times becoming agitated and more confused.

 What are the components of a comprehensive dysphasia assessment?

 What are the best practices to address dysphasia in the setting of advanced illnesses?

Definition and Causes

Dysphagia, defined as difficulty swallowing, is a common symptom for patients with life-limiting illness, such as head and neck cancer, neuromuscular disease, stroke, HIV/AIDS, and advanced dementia. A characteristic feature of the final phase of dementia is loss of interest in eating, dysphagia, or both. Occasionally these patients do not realize they are experiencing dysphagia because the symptoms can be subtle and change slowly over time. However, they have significant and specific oral care needs that must be addressed to treat and prevent dysphagia. The physiology of swallowing is complicated, changing as the anatomy throughout the oropharynx and thorax changes; consequently there are many areas where pathology can lead to manifestations of illness. **Table 5** lists some of the common conditions that interfere with eating and includes suggestions for possible interventions.

Table 5. Conditions That Interfere with Eating and Suggested Interventions

Condition	Intervention
Dentures	Ensure dentures are available and fit properly.
	Adjust or replace dentures if needed.
	Offer pureed foods.
Poor dental hygiene	Encourage brushing and flossing two to three times a day.
	Painful dental caries and broken teeth may need to be extracted.
Taste disorders	Treat sinusitis, thrush, or other infections.
	Provide supplemental vitamins including zinc[106] and other minerals (a stage III trial on high-dose zinc demonstrated equivocal benefit).[107]
Weakness or neuromuscular problems	Offer soft or pureed foods.
	Cut food into bite-sized pieces.
	Provide small, frequent meals.
	Moisten food with gravy, sauce, sour cream, or mayonnaise.
	Avoid hard, dry, or sticky foods.
	Help the patient into an upright position and stabilize her head.
	Use aids for easier drinking and eating (eg, a drinking glass with a cut-out for the nose).
	Use crushed, liquid, or rectal suppository forms of medications.
	Encourage the patient to chew thoroughly and to remain upright for 15 minutes after eating.
Stress and tension	Provide a calm, unhurried environment.

It is helpful to think of the causes of dysphagia as either neurologic or nonneurologic in origin (see **Table 6**). This approach will aid in the differential diagnosis when evaluating patients and will help determine how extensive the evaluation needs to be. When dysphagia initially presents as difficulty swallowing solids and then progresses to difficulty swallowing liquids, the cause is often obstructing lesions. When dysphagia for solids and liquids occurs almost simultaneously, neuromuscular disorders are frequently the cause.

Swallowing problems are common in palliative care, and data show that in the palliative phase the incidence of swallowing problems can be as high as 79%. These difficulties result in discomfort for the patient and raise concern for the caregiver.[109]

In addition, when rating symptoms of dysphagia, relatives and family members of the person who is dying may rate it as equally distressing as other symptoms at the end of life, whereas nursing staff responses suggest they only correlate loss of appetite with swallowing problems.

Assessment

Dysphagia is extremely common for people with advanced illness and can present subtly; therefore, a low index of suspicion and thorough history are imperative. When signs and symptoms of dysphagia become evident, the clinical history in conjunction with consideration of the differential diagnoses and overall prognosis will help clinicians delineate the most appropriate workup and management plan. The incidence of swallowing problems for patients with a noncancer diagnosis is reported to be higher than for patients with cancer, especially in the context of neurological illnesses such as stroke, ALS, and dementia.

Table 6. Neurologic and Other Causes for Dysphagia

Neurologic Causes	Other Causes
Stroke	Head and neck cancer
Amyotrophic lateral sclerosis	Mucosal injury (eg, prolonged endotracheal intubation)[108]
Parkinson's disease	Medications
Poliomyelitis	• Large pill size (potassium chloride)
Multiple sclerosis	• Nonsteroidal antiinflammatory drugs
Myasthenia gravis	Pharmacologic effect
Myopathies	Antibiotics (doxycycline, trimethoprim/sulfamethoxazole)
	• Anticholinergics
	• Angiotensin-converting enzyme inhibitors
	• Antihistamines
	Gastroesophageal reflux disease
	Status postchemotherapy or postradiation
	Esophageal cancer
	Achalasia
	Scleroderma

The role of a speech-language pathologist is equally important to help assess the safety of oral intake. That is, the expertise and knowledge of speech-language pathologists in feeding and swallowing, cognition, and communication affords unique and relevant contributions to the care plans of people with advanced illness. That being said, providers need to remain cautious because some speech-language pathologists remain unfamiliar with the goals of palliative care and may inappropriately focus solely on risks rather than helping the patient and family identify the safest and most palatable diet. Importantly, the patient goals may override the "safest diet," which should be honored as part of patient autonomy and the individualized care plan. The diagnostic evaluation of the speech-language pathologist should also be tailored to the patient's condition. Goals with invasive procedures and repeat testing may be overly burdensome without an impact on the care plan; therefore, simple bedside testing may often be the favored approach. Finally, although knowledge of aspiration risk is important and may lead to a particular diet recommendation, the benefit-burden ratio of limiting dietary choices near the end of life is less likely to change the overall illness trajectory and may cause undue patient suffering.[110]

Management

Because conservative management can ameliorate dysphagia for a majority of patients with life-limiting illness, a comprehensive, interdisciplinary treatment plan should emphasize good oral hygiene and general measures that any member of the treating team can implement.[111] Each caretaker should be familiar with the treatment modalities listed in Table 5 to avoid deferring simple changes that can make a difference early on in patient care. In addition, involving speech and occupational therapy services can help with postural and adaptive techniques to limit dysphagia and aspiration risk. The interventions listed in **Table 7** may help palliative symptoms after a working diagnosis has been determined for more complicated etiologies.

Irreversible Dysphagia

When dysphagia is the result of esophageal obstruction or when it is irreversible and progressive, the practitioner and the interdisciplinary team should consider whether the patient is a suitable candidate for more invasive measures, such as

- surgical resection or laser ablation on an obstructing lesion
- palliative radiation therapy[127]
- placement of an esophageal stent[128,129] with or without brachytherapy[130] (it has been shown that stent placement alone is inferior to stent placement combined with brachytherapy for patients with advanced esophageal cancer).

These procedures, particularly esophageal dilation and stenting,[131] are useful when the prognosis is at least weeks or months. However, proceeding with these interventions can be burdensome and may not be consistent with the goals of care set by patients as their disease

Table 7. Dysphagia: Medical Causes and Pharmacologic Treatments

Condition	Suggested Pharmacologic Treatments
Dry mouth caused by radiation or disease	Consider mandibular salivary gland transfer or parotid-sparing radiation techniques for prevention[112,113]
	Pilocarpine, 5 mg to 10 mg three times per day, preferably initiated prior to radiation[114] (watch for troublesome respiratory secretions or diarrhea[115]); or cevimeline, 30 mg three to four times per day (watch for sweating, increased urgency/frequency of urination, increased nasal/lacrimal secretions, and joint pain) Note: Sialagogues generally need to be administered for the rest of a patient's life after radiation[115]
	Saliva substitute or oral gel every 1-2 hours or sugar-free gum[116]
	Pilocarpine combined with a saliva substitute
	Avoidance of glycerin swabs and lemon juice[117]
Dryness caused by medications	Reduced dosage of medication, if possible
	Change medication; for example, use metoclopramide or haloperidol instead of prochlorperazine or chlorpromazine, and use an SSRI or trazodone instead of amitriptyline[118]
	Fluoride to prevent dental damage
	Pilocarpine, 5 mg PO twice a day[119]
Oral candidiasis	Oral nystatin suspension, 10 mL to 15 mL four times a day, swish for a full 60 seconds and swallow[120] Note: Difficult for patients with taste changes because of exceedingly sweet taste of suspension
	Clotrimazole, 10 mg troches, one dissolved in the mouth five times daily (difficult for a patient with a dry mouth) or fluconazole, 100 mg one to two times daily, for 10-14 days (equally effective)
Bacterial infection (periodontal disease is most common)	Adequate oral hygiene and an antibiotic; chlorhexidine gluconate, 0.12% 30 mL swish and spit twice a day may palliate periodontal infection

Continued on page 26

Table 7. Dysphagia: Medical Causes and Pharmacologic Treatments *(continued)*

Condition	Suggested Pharmacologic Treatments
Viral infection	Acyclovir, 400 mg five times daily for 7-10 days for acute infection or 800 mg three times daily for chronic suppression; or valacyclovir, 500 mg twice daily for 3 days for acute infection or 500 mg to 1,000 mg daily for chronic suppression (evidence of superiority of one agent or dosing schedule is lacking)[121]
Reflux esophagitis	Proton pump inhibitor Placement of patient in a more upright position by using wedges or pillows or putting bricks under the head of the bed
Mucosal damage from other causes	Lidocaine 2%, 2 mL to 5 mL every 4-8 hours (can be diluted or flavored if desired); can cause aspiration if used before meals Combination mouthwash containing two or three of the following (little evidence to support; avoid alcohol-based rinses): • loperamide[122] • tetracycline • hydrocortisone Doxepin oral rinse 5 mL (25 mg/5 mL concentration) swish for 30-60 seconds up to four times a day[123] Tamine mouthwash (20 mg/5 mL) every 3-4 hours as needed[124] Topical opioids such as morphine mouthwash[125] Parenteral opioids
Dryness caused by systemic dehydration	Increase liquid intake orally, if possible; try frozen juice, flavored ice, or popsicles Try ice chips, atomizer, or sips of water; as death approaches, encourage family members to keep the patient's mouth moist with a few drops of water from a syringe or a moist sponge stick, which may relieve dry mouth more effectively than parenteral fluids;[126] this involves family members in the patient's care

PO, by mouth; SSRI, selective serotonin reuptake inhibitor

progresses. For patients with esophageal cancer, metal stenting is currently the main option to palliate malignant obstruction. Endoscopic gastrostomy may be a suitable enteral nutrition technique for patients unfit for esophageal stenting; it is consistent with the care goals and has an overall reported mean survival after percutaneous endoscopic gastrostomy (PEG)–tube insertion of 5.9 months.[132]

Role of Artificial Nutrition

Feeding often represents well-being and frequently becomes the focus of families and patients near the end of life. Preserving nutrition and daily functional capacity is a commonly cited goal along with relieving hunger and thirst, which may lead families to ask about the role of artificial nutrition.

If procedural interventions are not feasible or do not provide sustained relief, and prognosis is weeks or months, it may be appropriate to consider a gastrostomy tube. This may be discussed in cases in which hunger is present and ongoing nutrition is desired by the patient or family. Alternatively, a nasogastric (NG) tube is more temporary and much easier to insert but tends to be less tolerated in the long term and, because of smaller lumen, tends to clog more easily. Artificial nutrition appears to be beneficial in certain clinical settings, such as for patients with ALS[133] or who are in a persistent vegetative state.[134,135] In addition, a patient who is actively being treated for head and neck or esophageal cancer may benefit from artificial nutrition via PEG or NG tube.[135]

Beyond these scenarios artificial enteral nutrition has not shown qualitative results and does not prolong life.[136] Studies of patients with dementia and patients with advanced terminal stages of cancer indicate that artificial nutrition does not lead to benefits such as life prolongation, prevention of aspiration, or reduction of pressure sores.[135,137] Some studies suggest potential patient harms, particularly in dementia, including an increased likelihood of the development of pressure sores, increased healthcare utilization such as emergency department visits, and increased need for physical and chemical restraints.[138,139] Discussions regarding PEG tube insertion should take place in the early stages of the diagnosis of terminal conditions, dementia, or neuromuscular disease. Caregivers need to be educated regarding QOL feeding, hand feeding, assisted oral feeding, safest diet, and aspiration precautions.

When it comes to PEG versus NG tube feeding, studies have not revealed a difference in the outcomes of these two methods.[140] In the absence of such interventions, a trial of parenteral hydration may be appropriate to support and treat dehydration-related symptoms. However, parenteral nutrition should not be given regularly, and a thorough assessment needs to be done before the initiation of parenteral nutrition, including consideration of the patient's clinical condition, psychosocial aspects, and potential economic constraints. Hypodermoclysis (subcutaneous fluid infusion) is as effective as intravenous hydration and may be safer, less costly, and more comfortable.[141]

Patients with dysphagia are at high risk for aspiration, and aspiration pneumonia is a frequent complication. One study, which looked at Parkinson's disease and dysphagia trends over a 32-year period, revealed a tenfold increase in aspiration pneumonia and an associated increase in mortality.[142] At later stages of disease, patients may not be able to tolerate oral secretions, much less excess parenteral nutrition or hydration. Patients with gastrostomy are not immune to complications of aspiration.[140] Because aspiration may be a terminal event, it is prudent to discuss this with the patient and family and help them develop their goals of care regarding the use of antibiotics and supplemental nutrition and hydration in the event infections or complications occur.

Helping the family cope with feelings of anxiety and guilt about the patient's low intake may be the most important intervention. As always, involvement of the interdisciplinary team is essential, and ongoing discussions regarding realistic and appropriate goals of care are needed.

Anorexia-Cachexia

Clinical Situation

Silas and Carla

Silas is a 67-year-old man with colon cancer who is referred for hospice and palliative care. The primary concern voiced by Silas's family is his lack of appetite. Silas's wife, Carla, and his adult children are extremely upset because Silas is not eating. They are particularly worried because the dietitian at a regional cancer center told them that Silas needed to drink six cans of nutritional supplement every day or he would need a feeding tube. Silas says he just doesn't feel like eating, the supplements are not to his liking, and he does not want a feeding tube in his nose. His principal complaints are abdominal discomfort and increasing weakness.

A detailed history reveals that Silas's colon cancer was diagnosed 1 year ago, and he has documented metastases to his liver. He had received chemotherapy, but when the disease began to progress, the oncologist indicated that Silas was no longer a candidate for further anticancer treatment. For the past several months Silas has had a paracentesis approximately once a month for recurrent malignant ascites. His medications include oxycodone, 5 mg tablet every 4 hours as needed, which provides moderate pain relief. Silas is eating a few bites of soft food four times a day; however, despite his limited intake, his weight has decreased only 10 pounds during the past 30 days due to his increased ascites. Silas drinks fluids with his meals and sips water throughout the day. He has not had a bowel movement for 6 days.

The physical examination reveals a blood pressure of 90/60 mm Hg, a pulse of 100, and regular respirations at 18 breaths per minute. Silas's chest is clear to auscultation, his heart has a rapid but regular rate, and his abdomen is mildly distended with an enlarged, palpable liver in the right upper quadrant and moderate ascites. An examination of his oral mucosa reveals white patches on the palate, and he admits to some discomfort with swallowing. A rectal examination reveals a large amount of soft stool.

 What is an appropriate assessment of patients who experience anorexia?

 What pharmacologic interventions are helpful?

 What nonpharmacologic interventions should be considered?

Definition and Pathophysiology

Anorexia is a common complication of terminal illness, reflecting a metabolic, cytokine, and neuroendocrine-mediated cascade of events leading to a loss of appetite for food, usually resulting in cachexia.[143-145] An international panel of experts in 2011 defined cancer cachexia as a multifactorial syndrome defined by an ongoing loss of skeletal muscle mass (with or without loss of fat mass) that cannot be fully reversed by conventional nutritional support and leads to progressive functional impairment.[146] Its pathophysiology is characterized by a negative protein and energy balance driven by a variable combination of reduced food intake and abnormal metabolism. The generally agreed upon diagnostic criterion for cachexia includes weight loss greater than 5% or weight loss greater than 2% in individuals already showing reduction in body mass index or skeletal muscle mass within the past 6 months.[146]

Chronic medical conditions are frequently exacerbated by cachexia, and response to curative treatments wane. The prevalence of cancer-related cachexia is approximately 60% to 80% and more commonly experienced in gastric, pancreatic, colorectal, and lung cancer patients.[147] Cardiopulmonary conditions are also associated with cachexia, with prevalence reported at 25% to 35% and 5% to 15% for COPD and CHF, respectively. Liver and renal diseases are also associated with cachexia; rates can approach 50% for both.[147]

Cachexia, or disease-related muscle loss, is distinct from sarcopenia, or age-related[148,149] muscle loss. The metabolic relationships between these two conditions help distinguish them. Each condition is associated with decreased muscle protein synthesis, muscle mass, strength, and function, along with increased insulin resistance. Cachexia has an increase in the basal metabolic rate with inflammation and increased muscle degradation, whereas sarcopenia involves basal metabolic rate decreases with minimal inflammation or change in muscle degradation. At the same time, sarcopenia generally has an increase in fat composition and cachexia does not. Given these key differences, treatment approaches may differ and studies that demonstrate improvement in one condition may not apply to the other.

Starvation studies demonstrate a physiological shift of energy substrate from carbohydrates to fat with an associated increase in ketone bodies, diminished amino acid metabolism with a decrease in urea load and, ultimately, a decline in urine volume and the need for water.[150] These changes are reflected in what is seen clinically in patients with advanced anorexia—a decrease in appetite because of presence of ketones, a decrease in urine volume, and a lack of thirst.

Surprising to most families and physicians, cachexia is not a result of reduced nutritional intake and typically is unresponsive to supplemental nutrition.[151] Instead, the anorexia-cachexia syndrome is multifactorial. Studies have shown that chronic inflammation is key in the mechanism of wasting as indicated by the upregulation of lipolysis,[152] increased muscle-protein catabolism and decreased anabolism, increased resting energy expenditure, and an increase in acute-phase proteins and proinflammatory cytokines.[153]

As research into the cellular and molecular levels of anorexia-cachexia becomes more sophisticated, therapeutic methods to mitigate the severity and rapidity of this process in affected patients ideally will emerge.

Cachexia in cancer is associated with worse patient-related outcomes. Disease-specific differences for patients who have cachexia compared with those who do not include a poorer response to anticancer therapy and a shorter time to disease progression along with increased toxicity from such treatments.[154] Similarly, cancer cachexia is associated with decreased physical functioning, increased dependence in activities of daily living, increased healthcare utilization, particularly hospitalizations with longer lengths of stay, and a decreased QOL compared to patients without cachexia.[155]

Assessment

The clinician should focus on identifying treatable culprits contributing to anorexia-cachexia syndrome. A careful history and physical examination should always be performed, with emphasis on weight-loss history and symptoms of treatable physical conditions and associated psychosocial issues.

Etiology and Management

Impaired oral intake may be a consequence of secondary nutrition impact symptoms: dry mouth; taste or smell alterations; stomatitis; odynophagia; dysphagia; severe constipation or bowel obstruction; nausea and vomiting; and uncontrolled symptoms such as pain, depression, dyspnea, or delirium.[156]

Catabolic states may be induced by acute or chronic infections and potentially reversible metabolic abnormalities such as hyperthyroidism, B_{12} deficiency, adrenal insufficiency, and hypogonadism. A 2011 retrospective chart review of 151 patients at the MD Anderson Cancer Center's Cachexia Clinic in Houston, TX, revealed a median of three secondary nutrition impact symptoms per patient, with most commonly reported symptoms being early satiety (62%), constipation (52%), nausea or vomiting (44%), and mood changes (42%). A median of two interventions were recommended per patient, most commonly including metoclopramide for early satiety and nausea (79%), laxatives for constipation (87%), antidepressants for mood disorders (81%), and zinc for dysgeusia (48%). In addition, 4% of patients had hyperthyroidism, 3% had vitamin B_{12} deficiency, and 73% of men had hypogonadism. After receiving treatment for secondary nutrition impact symptoms and simple replacement therapy for metabolic abnormalities, statistically significant improvements in both appetite scores and weight gain (34%) were found in those who returned for follow up.[156]

A variety of iatrogenic events (related to certain medications, chemotherapy, and radiation) can exacerbate anorexia-cachexia. **Table 8** offers a mnemonic to help remember some of the culprits that contribute to anorexia-cachexia.

Table 8. Reversible Causes of Anorexia

A	Aches and pains	See *UNIPAC 3.*
N	Nausea and gastrointestinal dysfunction	See section on Nausea and Vomiting on page 43.
O	Oral candidiasis	See Table 7.
R	Reactive (or organic) depression or anxiety	See *UNIPAC 2.*
E	Evacuation problems (constipation, retention)	See the section on Bowel Obstruction on page 55 and *UNIPAC 3.*
X	Xerostomia (dry mouth)	See Table 7.
I	Iatrogenic (radiation, chemotherapy, or drugs)	Reconsider burdens and benefits of the therapy.
A	Acid-related problems (gastritis, peptic ulcers)	Consider a proton pump inhibitor or H_2 blocker.

Depression, anxiety, delirium, and dementia all can lead to anorexia-cachexia. Patients and families may experience such financial hardship that they may have to prioritize whether to purchase medications or food, which emphasizes the need for a psychosocial assessment by a trained social worker or other team member in the care of patients with advanced illness.

It also is important to recognize that anorexia can present as part of a symptom cluster that helps direct the patient history and physical along with management strategies. Three well-defined symptom clusters associated with anorexia include (a) early satiety, dyspepsia, nausea, and bloating; (b) depression, anxiety, and insomnia; and (c) nausea, fatigue, and pain. Based upon the symptom cluster, one can delineate a more specific management strategy. For example, early satiety, dyspepsia, nausea, and bloating may respond better to metoclopramide.[157] Depression, anxiety, and insomnia should trigger clinicians to consider an antidepressant such as mirtazapine.[158] Nausea, fatigue, and pain cluster supports management with an antiemetic and possibly steroids depending upon prognosis and care goals.[159]

In addition, anorexia-cachexia carries a particularly poignant impact on a patient's family and loved ones.[160] In almost every culture, food represents nurturing, love, and the sustaining of life. Many families focus heavily on their loved one's eating habits, even attempting to push or force food in an attempt to delay death. This can cause profound psychosocial distress and decreased QOL, further leading to conflict when patients have accepted the anorexia as part of their dying process.

The clinician may defuse such conflicts with compassionate education and may share the following observations:

- Anorexia is part of the disease process and a natural part of life coming to an end.
- The patient is not starving because starvation relates to the lack of needed calories.
- Patients can live comfortably for long periods on minimal food and water.
- Forcing food on the patient may cause discomfort, nausea, and aspiration with associated respiratory distress.
- Artificial nutrition and hydration has not been shown to prolong life and may even shorten it. This modality may also cause nausea and vomiting, aspiration, and pulmonary congestion because the body may not be able to tolerate the increased fluid load at end of life.

The clinician may suggest the following action plans for families or caregivers:

- Allow patients to be the guides to new eating habits. Let them choose favorite foods, how and when they are to be eaten, and how much will be eaten. Discuss food goals with patients.
- Offer easy-to-swallow foods such as soup, pudding, or ice cream.
- Liberalize dietary restrictions. In the last weeks or months of life, blood sugar control and salt intake may assume less importance, especially when patients are eating less food in general. Patients with diabetes should be allowed to enjoy their favorite sweets, and cardiac patients should eat their favorite salty food in moderate portions.
- Identify alternative nonfood methods of expressing love such as listening to music together, reading or telling stories, or giving gentle massages.

Appetite Stimulants

Cachexia progresses along a continuum from precachexia to cachexia and ultimately to refractory cachexia, with the preponderance of pharmacologic and nonpharmacologic interventions being evaluated in patients with refractory cachexia. Ideally the management of anorexia and cachexia is multimodal, with exercise and nutritional and pharmacologic treatments being incorporated to yield the most optimal outcome. To date, studies generally focus on pharmacologic interventions alone; future research should incorporate a broader approach.

Pharmacologic appetite stimulation may be considered when reversible causes of anorexia are not readily found or not fully resolved. A therapeutic trial can be started in select patients with anticipated, specific goals defined and a time frame discussed among the clinician, interdisciplinary team, patient, and family. Unfortunately the literature demonstrates limited efficacy for a variety of medications used for this purpose. If there is no demonstrated benefit at the end of the agreed-upon time frame, the medication should be discontinued. Keep in mind, however, that goals are relative; a patient with end-stage cancer may not gain weight with an appetite stimulant, but the stimulant may effectively relieve anorexia and allow the social pleasure of eating dinner with family and friends. Commonly used preparations and their evidence bases are described in the following section.

Megestrol Acetate[161]

The literature demonstrates that megestrol increases appetite and body weight for cancer and HIV patients by increasing fat and water retention but not lean muscle mass.[162] Doses of 160 mg to 1,600 mg have been used for patients with cancer, and 400 mg to 800 mg for patients with HIV/AIDS. Although many anecdotal reports show an increase in appetite and QOL scores, an analysis of the literature reveals that only 15% of patients treated experienced a weight gain of more than 5% above baseline.[163-165] QOL outcomes surrounding megestrol use remain mixed.

Consider a starting dose of 400 mg by mouth daily; if appetite has not improved within approximately 2 weeks, escalate to 600 mg to 800 mg per day. The oral suspension (40 mg/mL) is less expensive and more bioavailable than tablets, so it is the preferred formulation when prescribed. Megestrol acetate seems to have a longer length of response than corticosteroids and can also be better tolerated. Side effect profiles, however, include an increased risk for adrenal suppression, hypogonadism, and thromboembolism.[166,167] Given megestrol's muted therapeutic benefit and lack of robust QOL data, along with risk of harm, its use has mostly fallen out of favor. In fact, it is on the Beers Criteria list for medications to be avoided in older adults[168] because of its minimal benefits and real risk of harm—1 in 12 patients on average will gain weight while 1 in 23 will die.

Olanzapine

Olanzapine has been a drug of interest for anorexia and weight loss, given its known side effect of weight gain. Approved by the FDA as an antipsychotic, olanzapine is known to block multiple neurotransmitters, including dopaminergic, serotonergic, muscarinic, and histamine receptors. Its effects, particularly regarding dopaminergic and serotonergic receptors, may improve nausea and emesis, partly explaining its mechanism because it does not appear to modulate inflammatory mediators.[169] A 2010 study randomized 80 patients with anorexia and weight loss to either megestrol acetate, 800 mg per day, or 800 mg per day combined with olanzapine, 5 mg per day. Results showed a significant difference, favoring the group receiving olanzapine. For patients receiving combination megestrol acetate/olanzapine, 84% experienced weight gain of more than 5% (compared with 38% of those receiving megestrol acetate alone), 64% experienced an increase in appetite (compared with 5%), 54% had improvement in nausea (compared to 7%), and 59% cited improved QOL scores (versus 13%).[170] Like all antipsychotics, olanzapine carries a black box warning regarding increased risks of death in elderly patients with dementia (see Black Box Warnings for Antipsychotic Medications on page 67).

Corticosteroids

A review of randomized clinical trials reveals that corticosteroids have a temporary effect (up to 4-8 weeks in duration) on subjective appetite without any increase in body mass.[163] That said, corticosteroids can be beneficial during the final weeks of life, not only for appetite stimulation, but also to help control a multitude of other symptoms, including pain, nausea, fatigue, and pruritus.[171]

The efficacy among various steroids is thought to be equivalent, but dexamethasone is often used because of its minimal mineralocorticoid effects and ease of dosing regimen (usually 2 mg-8 mg by mouth daily). Equivalent prednisone dosing is usually 20 mg to 40 mg by mouth daily. The side-effect profile includes worsening hyperglycemia, insomnia, hypertension, fluid retention, gastritis, and delirium. However, the importance of aggressive glucose and blood pressure control in the final weeks of life is debatable, and dosing in the morning can help minimize insomnia or delirium.[166]

Eicosapentaenoic Acid

Eicosapentaenoic acid, an omega-3 fish oil, is available as a dietary supplement. Randomized clinical trials have confirmed that patients with cancer taking 3 g per day of this acid experience an increase in lean body mass.[163] The effect has been compared to that of megestrol acetate. More trials, however, suggest weight stabilization over weight gain and perhaps an increase in physical activity.[172] Adherence may be limited by the ability to swallow the capsules and tolerate the side effects of burping and dysgeusia.[166] A 2011 literature review concluded there is not enough evidence to justify its use, but side effects were rare and mild.[173]

Thalidomide

Thalidomide is an immunomodulatory drug that may affect inflammatory cytokines. Random clinical trials have shown greatest efficacy for patients with HIV/AIDS with cachexia (see *UNIPAC 9*); a dosage of 200 mg to 400 mg a day increased weight independent of any change in appetite. Small studies suggest an effect in cancer-related cachexia in some patients.[163,174]

Cannabinoids

Dronabinol, a synthetic tetrahydrocannabinol (THC), is approved by the FDA for anorexia associated with HIV/AIDS, but the evidence is mixed. Some studies show an improvement in appetite and mood, but the literature overall shows little evidence to support its use for weight gain.[163,175] If a trial is warranted, dosing of dronabinol, 2.5 mg orally twice daily, before lunch and dinner is recommended; onset of action is approximately 30 minutes. Dosing can be titrated as high as 20 mg daily in divided doses but usually is limited by side effects such as hypotension, ataxia, somnolence, dry mouth, gastroparesis, euphoria, poor concentration, or hallucinations.

States continue to pass medical marijuana laws to help patients better control refractory symptoms that include anorexia. The endocannabinoid system has increased our understanding of the actions of exogenous cannabis. Endocannabinoids appear to positively affect pain, muscle tone, mood state, appetite, and inflammation, among others.[176] Cannabis contains more than 100 different cannabinoids and may have the capacity for analgesia through neuromodulation in ascending and descending pain pathways, neuroprotection, and antiinflammatory mechanisms.[176] Unfortunately there is little research to guide the use of medical marijuana.[177] One randomized, blinded study comparing cannabis extract, THC, and placebo in 243 patients with advanced cancer and weight loss revealed no significant difference between the three arms for any of the primary outcomes: appetite, QOL, or cannabinoid-related toxicity.[178]

Ghrelin

Ghrelin is a novel growth hormone–releasing peptide that is secreted in the stomach and has endocrine, metabolic, and other functions. Anamorelin is a high affinity, selective ghrelin-receptor agonist with anabolic and appetite-stimulating effects.[179] These effects are partly mediated through transient increases in growth hormone and insulin-like growth factor. Two pivotal trials in advanced non-small cell lung cancer patients with cachexia demonstrate that anamorelin, 100 mg twice daily, compared with placebo improved lean body mass and body weight with treatment differences emerging by 3 weeks. However, a primary study outcome did not reveal differences between the two groups in grip strength or survival. Importantly, many of the study participants were receiving antitumor therapy, indicating the treatment is safe and effective in patients on active cancer treatment.[179] Anamorelin has not yet received FDA approval, and its role will continue to evolve over time.

Fatigue

Manuel and Carmen

Manuel is a 63-year-old man who was diagnosed with multiple myeloma 6 months ago after presenting to his primary care physician with progressively worsening lower back pain that frequently awoke him from sleep. Although an initial X ray was unrevealing, a contrast-enhanced computed tomography (CT) showed a well-defined osteolytic lesion involving the fifth lumbar vertebrae. A radiographic skeletal survey confirmed the presence of multiple lytic bone lesions within the lateral aspect of the S1 vertebral body, right iliac bone, and left iliac crest. Bone marrow aspirate confirmed the presence of less than 30% plasma cells. Manuel was started on systemic chemotherapy and was referred to radiation oncology for palliative radiation therapy. Despite treatment, his disease has progressed. Over the past several weeks, he has experienced weight loss, depressed mood, and fatigue. He is no longer able to work as a long-distance truck driver and has become increasingly reliant on his wife of 40 years, Carmen. Given his decline, Carmen elects to bring him in for evaluation. Further inquiry reveals that Manuel is depressed; however, this is situational and related to his poor prognosis. On physical examination, he is unable to stand from a seated position without two-person assistance. He is cachectic and pale. There is evidence of skin tenting. Laboratory testing reveals a hemoglobin of 8 g/dL and albumin-corrected calcium of 11.5 g/dL. He states that he is reluctant to take corticosteroids given his history of steroid-induced psychosis.

 What is the appropriate assessment of this patient's fatigue?

 What nonpharmacologic approaches can help?

 What pharmacologic interventions could be helpful?

Definition and Etiology

Fatigue is a persistent, subjective, unpleasant sense of physical, emotional, and/or cognitive tiredness or exhaustion related to a disease state or its treatment that interferes with ones' usual level of functioning.[180] Fatigue has several presentations, including generalized weakness, which manifests as difficulty initiating activity; easy fatigability in association with reduced capacity maintaining performance; mental fatigue causing impaired cognition; and emotional lability.[181] It is pervasive and has been commonly reported by patients with cancer as well as other serious illnesses, including multiple sclerosis, ALS, COPD, heart failure, HIV/AIDS, and renal failure.[182] With regard to prevalence, studies have shown that 48% to 75% of patients with cancer and upwards of 85% of patients with serious, life-threatening illnesses at the end of life experience fatigue.[183-185]

For many patients, fatigue is often cited as being among the most distressing symptoms because of its negative impact on QOL as well as functional status.[186] Furthermore, it can be a harbinger of worsening disease severity. Many of the pharmacological treatments used in palliative care, including antidepressants, benzodiazepines, opioids, muscle relaxants, and first generation antihistamines, cause fatigue.[187]

The pathophysiology of fatigue is complex because its manifestation is influenced by physiologic as well as psychosocial etiologies. Furthermore, evidence on symptom clusters suggests that fatigue is related to, and exacerbated by, other symptoms such as pain, dyspnea, nausea, anxiety, muscle spasticity, and decreased cognition.[188] Although there has been much interest in the interplay of the immune system and hormonal dysregulation with suppression of the hypothalamic-pituitary axis in the pathogenesis of fatigue, there is insufficient evidence to support a role for circulating cytokines; further research is needed.[189]

Assessment

A patient's history is the most important component of the evaluation for fatigue. The ESAS is a brief, practical, rapid, and visual validated instrument consisting of 11-point numerical rating scales for self-report of nine common symptoms in palliative care, with a 10th scale for a patient-specific symptom. This scale allows for the creation of a clinical profile of symptom severity over time, including pain, tiredness, nausea, depression, anxiety, drowsiness, appetite, well-being, and shortness of breath.[190]

Assessment should also include screening for psychiatric disorders, evaluation of sleep hygiene, nutritional/metabolic evaluation, activity assessment, and inventory of prescription as well as over-the-counter medications and illicit drug use. Extensive laboratory testing in the absence of pertinent historical positives are of little diagnostic utility.[191]

Management

Management of fatigue is cause-specific when conditions known to cause fatigue can be identified and treated. When a reversible cause is not readily identified, nonpharmacologic (eg, exercise therapy, nutrition, sleep therapy, psychosocial interventions) and pharmacologic (eg, hematopoietics, antidepressants, psychostimulants, steroids) strategies can be applied alone or in combination.[180,192]

Treatment of Reversible Causes

In many cases fatigue is multifactorial, which explains why this condition can be so difficult to treat. **Table 9** highlights several of the most notable causes of fatigue.

Nonpharmacologic Management

After reversible causes of fatigue have been either ruled out or treated, the next step to treating fatigue is to implement nonpharmacologic therapies, specifically education, exercise, and energy-conservation therapies. These interventions require a multidisciplinary team that assesses patients' fatigue levels regularly and systematically and incorporates education and counseling regarding strategies for coping with fatigue.[180]

Evidence suggests that aerobic exercise regimens are associated with significant reductions in cancer-related fatigue for patients with earlier stages of cancer.[203,204] Data, however, is inconclusive for resistance exercise.[203,205,206] A graduated exercise program beginning with more modest levels of physical activity that increases in intensity over time is preferred.[207] A simple regimen of walking, biking, low-impact aerobics, or swimming may improve energy levels and help with appetite, strength, self-image, and bowel habits.[208]

Exactly how physical activity reduces fatigue in advanced cancer populations is largely unknown; future investigations, including systematic reviews, will aim to address this quandary.[209]

Several studies exploring the efficacy of psychosocial intervention, or therapy aimed at addressing perpetuating factors for persistent fatigue (eg, dysfunctional cognitions concerning fatigue, adverse coping mechanisms, fear of recurrence, disruption of sleep and activity patterns), as well as instruction in energy conservation, physical activity, sleep hygiene, distress management, nutrition, and pain control, to manage cancer-related fatigue have shown reduced fatigue in the intervention group relative to controls.[210-212] Although data are limited, alternative interventions including mindfulness, yoga, and acupuncture may help in the management of cancer-related fatigue.[213]

Pharmacologic Management

When reversible causes of fatigue have been identified and treated and nonpharmacologic interventions have been tried and deemed ineffective, pharmacotherapy may be warranted. Multiple agents have been investigated, including acetyl-L-carnitine, donepezil, amantadine, pemoline, modafinil, dexamphetamine, paroxetine, fluoxetine, dexamethasone, methylprednisolone, medroxyprogesterone acetate, alfacalcidol, armodafinil, acetylsalicylic acid, mistletoe extract, and testosterone.[182] Fatigue research in palliative care has mostly focused on modafinil and methylphenidate. However, a 2015 *Cochrane* review concluded that there is insufficient evidence to support the use of a specific medicine to treat fatigue experienced by patients receiving palliative care.[182]

Table 9. Reversible Causes of Fatigue

Organ dysfunction/ failure	Cardiac, pulmonary, renal, or hepatic failure contribute to fatigue over time. This may be true especially for patients with end-stage organ failure such as congestive heart failure.
Endocrine dysfunction	Hypogonadism: This is common in men with cancer who are taking opioids[193]; consider testosterone replacement in men with testosterone levels lower than 200 ng/dL.[194,195]
	Hypothyroidism: Check thyroid-stimulating hormone and titrate thyroid replacement drugs as indicated.
	Diabetes mellitus: acute glycemic excursions, microvascular complications (eg, diabetic nephropathy, neuropathy), and macrovascular complications (eg, peripheral arterial disease) are associated with fatigue.[196]
Anemia	Consider transfusions: Anemia occurs in up to 50% of all patients with cancer, with multiple trials showing significant improvement in overall QOL with an increase in hemoglobin (usually more than 11-13 g/dL).[197]
	Although previous studies showed that erythropoietin and darbepoetin are effective for cancer-related fatigue, because of safety concerns and side effects shown by more recent studies, erythropoietin-stimulating agents should no longer be used.[182]
Malnutrition	See the section on Anorexia-Cachexia on page 29.
	Nutritional deficiency
Infection	Various types of infections have been associated with fatigue. It is presumed that infection induces impairment of immune memory, which may precipitate and perpetuate fatigue.[198]
Depression and anxiety	See *UNIPAC 2* for information about treatment of depression and anxiety.
	Consider adding a psychostimulant until longer-acting medications become therapeutic or if the prognosis is short. Testosterone may help some women.[199]
Pain	See *UNIPAC 3* for information about treatment of pain.
	Both pain and its treatment with opioids can contribute to fatigue. When opioids are thought to be contributing, try tapering the dose, rotating to a different opioid, or adding a low-dose stimulant.
Medications	Cease or adjust the dose of opioids, antidepressants, benzodiazepines, anticonvulsants, muscle relaxants, and first-generation antihistamines.

Continued on page 41

Table 9. Reversible Causes of Fatigue *(continued)*

Sleep disorder	Effective treatment of sleep disturbances includes managing cancer-related symptoms and implementing pharmacologic, nonpharmacologic (eg, provision of general sleep hygiene advice and discouraging over-sleeping), and environmental interventions.[200]
Electrolyte abnormalities	Electrolyte disturbances, including hypercalcemia and hypomagnesaemia, are associated with fatigue. Consider obtaining a metabolic panel and provide replacement and/or supplementation as appropriate.
Deconditioning	Exercise rehabilitation during or after curative or life-prolonging treatment is considered an effective means of restoring physical and psychological function.[201,202]

Methylphenidate

In a small clinical trial, methylphenidate, a stimulant best known for its treatment of attention deficit disorder, was shown to improve HIV/AIDS-related fatigue.[182] Several other low-quality studies show that methylphenidate is efficacious in management of cancer-related fatigue.[182] Meta-analysis of two of these studies comparing methylphenidate with placebo showed a slightly superior effect of methylphenidate.[214,215] Dosing recommendations vary, but for frail older adults, a generally accepted approach is to start a trial dose of 2.5 mg twice daily, generally administered first thing in the morning and at noon. If tolerated, one can titrate to more therapeutic dosages of 5 mg to 60 mg per day.

Modafinil

Modafinil, a central nervous system (CNS) stimulant known for treatment of narcolepsy, has been evaluated for patients with multiple sclerosis (MS).[216] A randomized, placebo-controlled, double-blind study by Stankoff and colleagues assessed whether modafinil is useful for fatigue for patients with MS. Modafinil was tested with 115 patients with MS, but results failed to demonstrate a superiority of modafinil over placebo.[217] A 2009 double-blind, placebo-controlled study conducted by Lange and colleagues investigated the effects of modafinil on focused attention, motor function, and motor excitability for patients with MS and fatigue.[218] Twenty-one patients were enrolled with a statistically significant improvement of fatigue as measured by symptom severity scales in the modafinil group versus placebo after 8 weeks of treatment.[218] Although a positive effect of treatment was observed, given the small sample size, the result must be interpreted with caution because meta-analysis of these two studies failed to demonstrate a significant effect.[182]

Of note, methylphenidate, not modafinil, is recommended in the 2017 National Cancer Center Network Guidelines for Cancer-Related Fatigue, but only after other reversible etiologies of fatigue are ruled out.[180]

A starting dose of modafinil is usually 100 mg to 200 mg in the morning, with doses over 200 mg rarely more effective and the lower dose usually being given to older adults.

Amantadine

Amantadine, an antiviral agent most commonly used for influenza, has been first-line treatment for MS-related fatigue, one of the most common and disabling symptoms in this population. Initial studies confirmed efficacy of amantadine for fatigue when compared with placebo.[219,220] A 2015 *Cochrane* review, however, revealed heterogeneous outcomes for amantadine efficacy in reducing MS-related fatigue when compared with placebo.[182]

Corticosteroids

Corticosteroids and hypothalamic-pituitary-adrenal axis dysfunction are implicated in the etiology of some symptom clusters in advanced cancer that include fatigue.[221,222] Data regarding its efficacy in treating fatigue are limited, however.[182] These drugs may have short-term benefit in treating fatigue and other symptom clusters near the end of life; unfortunately, long-term treatment can be limited by decreased efficacy and side-effect profile. Typical dosing for fatigue is dexamethasone, 1 mg to 2 mg orally twice daily, or prednisone, 5 mg to 10 mg orally twice daily; these doses can be titrated for efficacy and to limit side effects.[223] Side effects from corticosteroids may include elevations in blood pressure and glucose, upper gastrointestinal (GI) symptoms, agitation, insomnia, and delirium.

Erythrocyte-Stimulating Agents

The 2015 *Cochrane* review excluded agents including erythropoietin and darbepoetin from the analysis because their use is contraindicated due to safety concerns and side effects, including insomnia, delirium, anorexia, anxiety, confusion, tremor, and cardiac arrhythmias.[182,223]

Fluoxetine

A study consisting of 129 patients with MS showed that a treatment with fluoxetine, 20 mg daily for 12 weeks, resulted in improved functional and depression scores when compared with placebo.[224]

Other Therapies

Studies investigating dextroamphetamine, donepezil, paroxetine, testosterone, pemoline, Acetyl-L-carnitine, alfacalcidol, armodafinil, and acetylsalicylic acid either revealed modest effect or did not show a positive effect on management of fatigue when compared with placebo.[182] In the case of acetylsalicylic acid, two studies showed a statistically significant improvement of fatigue, but no definitive conclusion could be drawn because varying doses were used.[182] The clinical use of mistletoe extract, megestrol acetate, and medroxyprogesterone acetate warrant additional studies to better demonstrate their clinical efficacy.[182]

Nausea and Vomiting

Clinical Situation

Sookie and Guy

Sookie is a 52-year-old woman who lives with her husband Guy. Two years ago Sookie was diagnosed with metastatic cervical cancer. She received several rounds of chemotherapy, but the cancer continued to spread. A recent computed tomography (CT) scan shows peritoneal carcinomatosis. Sookie's oncologist has been keeping her comfortable with oxycodone/acetaminophen 5 mg/325 mg, one tablet every 4 hours as needed. One to two tablets a day had been keeping her pain adequately controlled, and she had been sleeping well at night. Over the past 3 weeks her pain has worsened greatly, so 1 week ago her oncologist started long-acting morphine, 30 mg twice a day, and short-acting morphine, 15 mg every 4 hours as needed. Sookie's pain is much improved with the morphine, but after a few days she has developed nausea, and yesterday she vomited for the first time. She has small, round bowel movements every 2-3 days. Her current medications are

- morphine extended release, 30 mg orally twice a day
- short-acting morphine, 15 mg orally every 4 hours as needed (once a day)
- senna, 1 tablet at bedtime
- ibuprofen, 400 mg orally every 6 hours as needed (2-3 times a day).

When Sookie returns to the oncologist, she is tired from lack of sleep. On physical examination, her abdomen is mildly distended, but she does not appear to have ascites. Although she is experiencing generalized abdominal discomfort, she reports no specific area of abdominal pain. She reports that she feels the urge to urinate frequently but can pass only small amounts of urine each time. A rectal examination reveals soft stool and mild tenderness in the rectal area.

Sookie's oncologist rotates from the short- and long-acting morphine and starts fentanyl, 25 mcg patch every 72 hours, and hydromorphone, 2 mg to 4 mg orally every 4 hours as needed for pain. She adds polyethylene glycol at night and stops the ibuprofen. Three days later, Guy calls the oncologist's office to report that Sookie's nausea has resolved. She is eating well and feels much better.

Six weeks later, Sookie is feeling much worse. Guy calls the oncologist and reports that Sookie's nausea is constant and she is vomiting two to three times a day. She is having trouble keeping down food and medications. Her pain has also worsened, but because she often vomits after taking her breakthrough pain medications, it is unclear if she needs to increase her opioids. She reports regular soft bowel movements with her current bowel regimen.

 What are potential contributors to the patient's nausea and vomiting?

 What pharmacologic and nonpharmacologic approaches to nausea and vomiting are effective?

Prevalence

Nausea and vomiting are relatively common symptoms with a variety of causes in terminally ill populations. In one study nearly 60% of terminally ill patients with cancer reported nausea, and 30% of these patients experienced vomiting.[225] The prevalence of nausea and vomiting is as high as 71% among patients with ovarian cancer, a disease commonly associated with obstructive symptoms.[226] In a cross-sectional national survey of 1,500 patients with cancer treated with chemotherapy or radiation therapy, 49% reported nausea or vomiting.[227] These symptoms often cause significant distress, but they can usually be controlled with targeted interventions for a majority of patients with advanced and end-stage illness.[228]

Pathophysiology

The vomiting reflex is activated by a cluster of neurons in the medulla known as the vomiting center. The vomiting center receives input directly from the cerebral cortex, sensory organs, and the vestibular apparatus in the inner ear. Anxiety and subsequent anticipation of nausea are common cortical triggers. Certain sights, smells, agitated motions, and brain tumors can act as sensory or vestibular triggers.

In addition, indirect stimulation of the vomiting center arrives from the chemoreceptor trigger zone located in the floor of the fourth ventricle, which lacks a true blood-brain barrier. The chemoreceptor trigger zone senses fluctuations in the concentration of various substances in the bloodstream,[229] primarily medications and their rate of uptake, metabolic disturbances, and signals from the GI tract. The chemoreceptor trigger zone stimulates the vomiting center with neurotransmitters such as serotonin, dopamine, acetylcholine, and histamine. Consequently, any therapeutic interference with these transmitters will prevent or mitigate activation of the vomiting center.

See **Figure 2** for a visual representation of the pathophysiology of nausea and vomiting.

Assessment

As with all symptoms, the clinician should take a careful history and perform a focused physical examination to identify specific physical and psychosocial contributors to nausea

Figure 2. Pathophysiology of Nausea and Vomiting

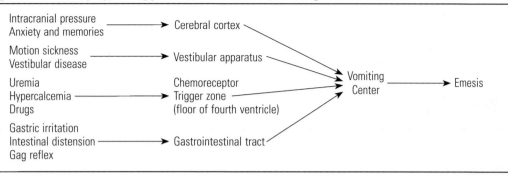

and vomiting. Common causes of nausea and vomiting in a palliative care population include chemical abnormalities (metabolic, drugs, and infections), impaired gastric emptying,[230] and visceral and serosal causes including constipation. Moreover, easily reversible causes can often be identified, particularly medications (notably opioids and constipation).[231] A useful mnemonic for the different causes of nausea and vomiting is "A VOMIT," illustrated below. **Table 10** offers a more comprehensive guide to etiology and treatment based on symptoms, and **Table 11** provides general pharmacologic guidelines for treating nausea and vomiting.

A Anxiety or anticipatory

V Vestibular

O Obstructive

M Medications/metabolic

I Infection/inflammation

T Toxins

Management

General Measures

Nausea and vomiting are debilitating symptoms for patients and exhausting for patients and families alike. Not only do they affect patients' ability to take their medications, but limited oral intake often leads to dehydration, electrolyte abnormalities, and weight loss, which cause a multitude of other complications. These complications interfere with therapies and social interaction and cause a significant amount of psychosocial distress.

Eating is usually problematic for patients who are experiencing nausea or vomiting. To minimize further symptoms, meals should be small, frequent, and consist of food the patient desires. This usually means avoiding foods with strong odors or unpleasant tastes. The patient should also drink frequent, small sips of fluids.

Table 10. Causes and Treatments of Nausea and Vomiting

Cause	Symptoms	Possible Treatment
Cortical		
Tumor in CNS or meninges	Neurologic signs or mental status problems	Dexamethasone Consider radiation therapy for new metastases.
Increased intracranial pressure	Projectile vomiting, headache	Dexamethasone
Anxiety, other conditioned responses	Anticipatory nausea, predictable vomiting	Counseling Benzodiazepines (eg, lorazepam)
Uncontrolled pain	Pain and nausea	Opioids, other pain medications, adjuvants
Vestibular/Middle Ear		
Vestibular disease	Vertigo or vomiting after head motion	Meclizine, 25 mg PO twice a day ENT consultation as appropriate
Middle-ear infections	Ear pain or bulging tympanic membrane	Antibiotic and/or decongestant, as appropriate
Motion sickness	Travel-related nausea	Scopolamine topical, 1.5 mg patch every 3 days Dimenhydrinate, 50 mg-100 mg PO every 4 hours (max 400 mg/day)
Chemoreceptor Trigger Zone		
Medications (eg, opioids, digoxin, chemotherapy, antibiotics, theophylline)	Nausea worse after medication is initiated and is exacerbated by increased dosage	Decrease medication dosage or discontinue medication, if possible
Metabolic (eg, renal or liver failure or tumor products)	Increased BUN, creatinine, bilirubin	Haloperidol, 0.5 mg-1 mg PO/SC every 4 hours as needed
Hyponatremia	Confusion, low sodium	Fluid restriction Demeclocycline
Hypercalcemia	Somnolence, delirium, high calcium	Hydration and pamidronate Dexamethasone

Table 10. Causes and Treatments of Nausea and Vomiting *(continued)*

Cause	Symptoms	Possible Treatment
Gastrointestinal Tract		
Irritation by medications (use of NSAIDs, iron, alcohol, antibiotics)		Stop drug, if possible Add proton pump inhibitor, misoprostol, or H_2 blocker
Tumor infiltration, radiation therapy to the GI tract, or infection (candida esophagitis, colitis, history of radiation therapy)		Promethazine, hydroxyzine Treatment of infection Serotonin 5-HT3 receptor antagonists, ondansetron
Constipation or impaction	Abdominal distension, long time since last bowel movement	Laxative Manual disimpaction if needed Enema
Incomplete obstruction by tumor or poor motility	Constipation unrelieved by treatment with motility agent	Metoclopramide
Tube feedings	Abdominal distension, diarrhea	Reduce feeding volume or discontinue feeding
Gag reflex from feeding tube	Vomiting after NG-tube insertion	Remove tube
Nasopharyngeal bleeding	Hemoptysis, epistaxis Blood visible in pharynx	Packing Vitamin K, if appropriate Sedation
Thick secretions	Cough-induced vomiting	Nebulized saline expectorant if strong cough reflex Anticholinergic if poor cough reflex

BUN, blood urea nitrogen; CNS, central nervous system; ENT, ear, nose, and throat; GI, gastrointestinal; NG, nasogastric; NSAIDs, nonsteroidal anti-inflammatory drugs; PO, by mouth; PRN, as needed; SC, subcutaneous.

Table 11. Antiemetic Guide: Pharmacologic Management[232]

Class of Drug	Initial Dose[A]		Comments[B]
	Oral	Parenteral	
Prokinetic Agents			
Metoclopramide	0.1 mg-0.15 mg/kg/dose (typically 5 mg-15 mg in adults) before meals and at bedtime, up to 60 mg/day	SC/IV = PO	Has both a dopamine blockade and some 5-HT3 receptor antagonist activities at higher doses. Primarily used for gastric stasis and GI dysmotility from various causes. May cause dystonia, which is reversible with diphenhydramine, 1.0 mg/kg. Antiemetic dosage is higher than prokinetic dosage by 0.1 mg-0.2 mg/kg/dose. Well tolerated with SC administration.
Antihistamines			
Useful for vestibular and gut receptor nausea and vomiting but relatively contraindicated for constipation because they further slow bowels. Anticholinergic properties may cause problems for older adults.			
Diphenhydramine	1 mg/kg/dose PO every 4 hours to a maximum of 100 mg/dose	SC/IV = PO	
Hydroxyzine	0.5 mg/kg-1.0 mg/kg/dose every 4 hours to a maximum of 600 mg/day	IM = PO	SC or IV extravasation can cause sterile abscess or tissue damage
Promethazine	0.125-0.5 mg/kg/dose (typically 25 mg) every 4 hours	IM/PO = PR	Use promethazine with caution; can cause dystonia (phenothiazine derivative). Can cause severe tissue damage if extravasates from IV

Table 11. Antiemetic Guide: Pharmacologic Management[232] *(continued)*

| Class of Drug | Initial Dose[A] | | Comments[B] |
	Oral	Parenteral	
Dopamine Antagonists			
Useful for medication and metabolic-related nausea and vomiting.			
• Can cause dystonia; reversible with diphenhydramine, 1 mg/kg, or benzatropine, 0.02 mg/kg-0.05 mg/kg/dose to a maximum of 4 mg IV.			
• IV can cause postural hypotension, QTc prolongation.			
• Give IV slowly.			
Haloperidol	0.5 mg-1.5 mg/dose every 6-12 hours, up to 5 mg twice daily IV/SC For children, 0.01-0.05 mg/kg/dose up to every 8 hours	SC/IV = ½ PO	Use with care; only some preparations can be given IV Use D5W to dilute Well tolerated with SC administration
Chlorpromazine	0.5 mg/kg-1 mg/kg (typically 10 mg-25 mg, up to 50 mg) every 8 hours	IV = PO	Very sedating Irritating to tissues with SC administration IV administration should be over 15-30 minutes to avoid hypotension
Prochlorperazine	0.2 mg/kg/dose every 4 hours to a maximum of 10 mg/dose	IV = PO	Irritating to tissues with SC administration
Olanzapine	2.5 mg-10 mg daily	PO	Works at multiple receptors Can cause somnolence and weight gain (with hyperglycemia)

Continued on page 50

Table 11. Antiemetic Guide: Pharmacologic Management[232] (continued)

Class of Drug	Initial Dose[A]		Comments[B]
	Oral	Parenteral	
Serotonin 5-HT3 Receptor Antagonists			
Also useful for postoperative and radiation-induced nausea and vomiting and as second- or third-line agents after other types of antiemetics have demonstrated limited utility or tolerability unless serotonin pathways thought to be involved			
Ondansetron	0.15 mg/kg/dose every 6 hours to a maximum of 8 mg/dose	SC/IV = PO	Particularly helpful in chemotherapy-induced nausea and vomiting; generic tablets available
			Side effects can include headache, dizziness, arrhythmias (due to QTc prolongation), and nervousness
			With IV metoclopramide, there is an increased risk of cardiac dysrhythmia
Granisetron	1 mg every 12 hours in adults	0.01 mg/kg-0.02 mg/kg every 8 hours	Particularly helpful in chemotherapy-induced nausea and vomiting
	0.04 mg/kg/dose in children; not approved for children younger than 2 years		
NK₁ Receptor Antagonists			
Aprepitant	125 mg on day 1, followed by 80 mg daily	PO	Particularly helpful in delayed chemotherapy-induced nausea and vomiting
Benzodiazepines			
Diazepam	0.05 mg/kg-0.2 mg/kg/dose every 6 hours (PO/PR)	PO/PR = IV	Helpful for anticipatory nausea and vomiting
	Patients younger than 5 years: max dose 5 mg; patients older than 5 years: max dose 10 mg		Diazepam stings during IV administration; use a large vein and dilute solution
Lorazepam	0.03 mg/kg-0.05 mg/kg/dose every 6 hours to a maximum of 4 mg/dose	IV = PO/SL	shorter half-life, no active metabolites
			Evidence mainly supports use for anticipatory nausea.

Table 11. Antiemetic Guide: Pharmacologic Management[232] *(continued)*

Class of Drug	Initial Dose[A]		Comments[B]
	Oral	Parenteral	
Corticosteroids			
Dexamethasone	6 mg-10 mg loading dose, then 2 mg-4 mg one to four times a day for maintenance	IM/IV = PO	Helpful for hepatic capsular distension, anorexia, and increased intracranial pressure
	If the patient weighs less than 10 kg, 1 mg/kg loading dose, then 0.1-0.2 mg/kg/dose two to four times a day for maintenance		Beware of long-term side effects Observe the patient for mood swings
Prednisone	1.5 mg dexamethasone = 10 mg prednisone	N/A	
Cannabinoids			
Dronabinol	2.5 mg two to four times a day to a maximum of 20 mg/day	N/A	Can cause dysphoria, drowsiness, or hallucinations Evidence for chemotherapy-induced nausea and vomiting
Other Anticholinergics			
Scopolamine Hydrobromide	Transdermal preparation: 1.5 mg changed every 72 hours	0.006 mg/kg/dose every 6 hours IV/SC	Helpful for motion- or movement-related nausea and vomiting Well tolerated by SC tissues Often causes dry mouth and blurred vision and sometimes causes confusion/sedation

D5W, 5% dextrose in water; GI, gastrointestinal; IM, intramuscular; IV, intravenous; PO, by mouth; PR, per rectum; SC, subcutaneous; SL, sublingual.

[A]*Doses are simply guidelines for initial dosing, as are the intervals (given as the shortest time) between initial dosing. Dose and interval can be titrated to relief of symptoms and side effects. May be given on an as-needed or scheduled basis.*

[B]*Many antiemetics are available; careful consideration of cost is important, especially near discharge. Affordability becomes equally important as efficacy in helping patients obtain all their necessary prescriptions. Most of the medications listed here are available as generic formulations with relatively lower cost per month with the exception of the newer 5-HT3 and NK1 receptor antagonists and dronabinol.*

Medications should be taken when best tolerated, either spread throughout the day or after meals. Antiemetics may be most effective if used prophylactically (on a regular schedule) in situations in which nausea may be expected to occur or recur.

Relaxation techniques are useful adjuncts to control symptoms, especially when anxiety is a significant contributor. The interdisciplinary team should address all nonphysical factors—psychological, social, and spiritual—that may exacerbate symptoms.

General management techniques and pharmacologic therapies are often initiated based on the presumed etiology of nausea and vomiting. This mechanistic approach involves determining the presumed pathway and receptor(s) involved and then using the most potent antagonist for treatment. The evidence to support the superiority of this approach over empiric treatment, which involves choosing an antiemetic to start (usually a dopamine antagonist or a serotonin 5-HT3 receptor antagonist), is weak. Although some causes (GI dysmotility, bowel obstruction) demonstrate greater response to targeted therapies, nausea etiology is often multifactorial. In addition, many drugs work across multiple receptors, likely contributing to the success of an empiric approach to treatment.[232]

A 2015 systematic review of the literature for treatment of nausea and vomiting in palliative care revealed a limited evidence base, with most of the studies involving patients with cancer. More high-quality randomized controlled trials of antiemetics are required that stratify cases on the basis of likely etiology. Ultimately the evidence base is limited, which makes it difficult to establish guidelines for antiemetics.[233]

Management of Persistent Nausea and Vomiting

If nausea and vomiting persist despite appropriate interventions, the patient should be reassessed. New or unappreciated etiologies may come to light and need to be treated separately.

A combination of antiemetics in different classes (see Table 11) may be necessary for certain patients or certain etiologies. For example, gastric decompression with an NG tube may be warranted in cases of gastric outlet obstruction, along with the use of octreotide or an anticholinergic to reduce GI fluid volumes. Metoclopramide may be warranted for stimulation of peristalsis, and dexamethasone may be recommended to reduce peritumor inflammation and swelling (see Bowel Obstruction on page 55 for more details). Other critical pathologies such as obstructive renal failure may require a procedural intervention for effective relief of symptoms.

Chemotherapy-Induced Nausea and Vomiting

One of the most challenging problems is chemotherapy-induced nausea and vomiting, which is markedly underestimated by treating physicians and often causes serious complications. These include failure to comply with cancer-therapy regimens; weight loss and malnutrition, which lead to difficulty fighting infections; and diminished QOL. Considering the numerous possibilities for chemotherapeutic regimens and that each agent acts by different mechanisms, it is understandable that no one regimen is universally effective; however, consensus guidelines are regularly updated. These classify neoplastic agents by emetic risk as either high, moderate, low, or minimal. The National Comprehensive Cancer Network updates their guidelines annually on the prevention and treatment of chemotherapy-induced nausea and vomiting, depending on the emetic risk of an agent.[234]

Generally, chemotherapy-induced nausea and vomiting can be divided into three distinct types: acute, delayed, and anticipatory.[235]

Acute
Acute nausea and vomiting occurs within 24 hours of chemotherapy, usually starting within 1 to 2 hours and peaking within 4 to 6 hours. Treatment can be administered with any of the usual agents, but a 2010 *Cochrane* review confirms that antiserotonergics (ondansetron, granisetron) have shown benefit for this indication.[235,236]

Delayed
Delayed nausea and vomiting occur after 24 hours, usually peaking within 48 to 72 hours and subsiding after 2 to 3 days. This type seems to be most common with agents such as cisplatin, carboplatin, cyclophosphamide, and other anthracyclines.[237] Often, delayed nausea does not respond as well to antiserotonergic or antidopaminergic agents.[238] Instead, antineurokinins (NK$_1$ receptor antagonists such as aprepitant) have shown a better effect on this syndrome when used in combination with a serotonin inhibitor and dexamethasone.[239]

Anticipatory
Anticipatory nausea is often the most challenging to address because it is a conditioned response to previous experiences, not mediated by neurotransmitters, and not as responsive to agents affecting these transmitters.[240] It is best to avoid the development of anticipatory nausea by aggressively and proactively treating nausea in this setting. After this type of chemotherapy-induced nausea and vomiting is established, however, psychotherapy focusing on cognitive-behavioral techniques and benzodiazepines have been most useful.

There is limited data for alternative medicines for symptomatic relief. Peppermint oil and ginger can be effective for some patients.[241]

Alternative Routes of Medication Delivery
If a patient is unable to swallow or retain oral formulations, other routes often are used in the palliative care setting that may be beneficial both in the interim (until nausea can be controlled) and at the end of life. Although intravenous line placement may be possible, similar dosing can be delivered subcutaneously, which is often less burdensome for patients and clinicians than obtaining IV access or giving intramuscular injections and can be done in both hospitals and at home with hospice (**Table 12**). Of note, the maximum tolerated hourly rate of a subcutaneous infusion is typically 3 mL/hour, necessitating careful evaluation of the concentration of the medication infused. Additional routes of administration, including sublingual, intranasal, and rectal, also should be considered.

Table 12. Palliative Medications Commonly Administered Subcutaneously

Drug	Indication	Comments
Dexamethasone	Anorexia, fatigue Elevated ICP, seizures Fever Nausea, vomiting Pain	Current practice: intermittent SC injection (SC use not recommended by the manufacturer) Administer slowly; may cause local burning, irritation
Fentanyl citrate	Dyspnea Pain	Current practice: both intermittent SC injection and CSCI (SC use not addressed by the manufacturer) Preferred in renal failure
Furosemide	Edema, ascites Pulmonary congestion	Onset of action about 30 minutes (compared to 5 minutes IV), duration of action about 4-6 hours Administer slowly or by CSCI[76] because of potential for local burning
Glycopyrrolate	Secretions Bowel obstruction	Current practice: intermittent SC injection and CSCI (SC use not addressed by the manufacturer) Doesn't cross the blood-brain barrier (limits sedation)
Haloperidol lactate	Agitation Delirium Nausea, vomiting	Current practice: intermittent SC injection (SC use not recommended by the manufacturer) SC or IV routes may increase risk of arrhythmias
Hydromorphone	Dyspnea Pain	Current practice: both intermittent SC injection and CSCI (SC use not addressed by manufacturer) Administer slowly; may cause pain, local irritation
Metoclopramide	Nausea, vomiting	SC use reported (not addressed by the manufacturer)
Midazolam	Anxiety Sedation	Current practice: intermittent SC injection (SC use not recommended by the manufacturer) Recommend a separate line for CSCI
Morphine sulfate	Dyspnea Pain	May have accumulation of metabolites in renal failure
Naloxone	Opiate overdose	Onset of action about 2-5 minutes (compared to 1-2 minutes IV)
Octreotide	Bowel obstruction GI bleeding	Current practice: intermittent SC injection Administer slowly; may cause stinging

CSCI, continuous subcutaneous infusion; GI, gastrointestinal; ICP, intracranial pressure; IV, intravenous; SC, subcutaneous

Note. Dosing all equivalent to IV dosing.

Bowel Obstruction

Clinical Situation

Marcel and Kasey

Marcel is 72 years old and has a history of stage IV colon cancer status postresection of primary tumor more than 1 year ago. His wife, Kasey, brings him to the clinic because Marcel has refused to eat for 2 days and has had worsening abdominal pain, nausea, and abdominal distention. Marcel has had chronic pain since his surgery that has been treated with a low dose of morphine (15 mg orally twice daily), but this pain has significantly increased over the past 2 days, now with a continuous and colicky component. Kasey tries to keep track of all the medications he is using, but she is not certain about how much morphine he has needed for breakthrough pain in the last day and is unsure about the timing of his last bowel movement.

On physical examination Marcel's abdomen is slightly distended with decreased bowel sounds and mild discomfort to diffuse palpation. A rectal exam reveals some firm stool in the rectal vault.

He is placed back on a bowel regimen. Marcel's symptoms improve. But several months later, he notices worsening abdominal swelling, followed by similar crampy abdominal pain, nausea, and vomiting. A review of his history reveals Marcel is taking all his medications, including the bowel regimen as prescribed, but he has not had a bowel movement in 4 days. Kasey brings him back to clinic, requesting "the constipation shot."

On physical exam Marcel has some temporal wasting but has gained a couple of pounds since his last visit. He appears uncomfortable with a distended abdomen, now with a mild fluid wave. Bowel sounds are decreased but an occasional tinkling sound is heard. A rectal exam reveals only mild soft stool in the vault, and Marcel confirms that although he has had no bowel movement, he does continue to occasionally pass gas.

 From what invasive procedures (such as surgery) do patients with bowel obstruction benefit?

 What is the best approach to the medical management of bowel obstruction?

Definition and Incidence

Bowel obstruction is the mechanical or functional blockage of the progression of food and fluids through the GI tract, causing nausea, vomiting, and abdominal pain. Incidence of bowel obstruction ranges between 5.5% and 42% for patients with ovarian cancer and between 10% and 28.4% for patients with colorectal malignancies.[242] Although bowel obstruction is most often a manifestation and complication of malignancy or treatment (such as surgical adhesions or postradiation fibrosis), other conditions can serve as the cause, such as severe fecal impaction from opioid use, inflammatory bowel disease, or benign growths.[242]

Etiology and Pathophysiology

With malignancy there may be an extension of a tumor directly into the bowel wall and lumen, adjacent carcinomatosis impinging on the bowel, or adherence of the tumor to the bowel wall with kinking of the bowel loop.[243] Regardless of etiology, bowel obstruction leads to hypoxia in the bowel wall and bacterial overgrowth, resulting in rising vasoactive intestinal peptide levels, which stimulate hypersecretion and splanchnic vasodilation.[244,245] Consequently the bowel distends proximally to the obstruction with a compensatory increase in peristalsis, leading to colicky abdominal pain and abdominal distension. The increased volume of intestinal secretions without adequate forward flow often leads to nausea and vomiting, which may be episodic or continuous.

In late stages of bowel obstruction, volumes of fluids and electrolytes may be substantial enough to sequester in the gut wall, leading to systemic hypotension and multiple organ failure. Bacterial overgrowth may lead to sepsis.[243]

Assessment

Bowel obstruction rarely occurs as an acute event. It usually develops as a late manifestation of advanced abdominal or pelvic malignancy.[246] Obstruction may be partial or complete and can result from benign causes such as adhesions or inflammatory bowel disease.

Physical signs include abdominal distention, visible peristalsis, and intermittent *borborygmus,* classically described as "rushes and tinkles." Complete bowel obstruction presents with *obstipation,* defined as a total lack of flatus or feces. Incomplete bowel obstruction presents with similar symptoms on an intermittent basis, including episodic passage of flatus and feces.

A diagnosis of obstruction can be made by conducting a careful history and physical examination. Upper GI obstructions are typically associated with early-onset nausea and vomiting with larger volumes of emesis. Nausea usually persists continuously or subsides only briefly after each episode of vomiting. In comparison, lower GI obstructions usually result in less pronounced and more episodic symptoms. Emesis will likely be bilious, and bacterial liquefaction of stool proximal to rectosigmoid obstructions (usually found in fecal impaction) may lead to liquid stool flowing around the lesion, presenting as diarrhea.

When the clinician suspects bowel obstruction, careful abdominal and digital rectal examinations should be performed. When the diagnosis is not clearly evident, plain abdominal radiographs usually are sufficient for further clarification. In a few cases, oral contrast studies may be useful to better visualize location and extent of obstruction. When malignant bowel obstruction is suspected or known, computed tomography (CT) scanning provides more information for prognostication and treatment planning.

Management

Constipation, Fecal Impaction

When obstructive symptoms are the result of fecal impaction, they are treatable with aggressive manual disimpaction, oral laxatives, suppositories, or enemas.

Astute clinicians will look for possible reversible underlying causes and exacerbating factors that may contribute to constipation. Patients with progressive disease often have limited or loss of mobility, underlying diseases that may impact gut motility and rectal tone/sensation, and multiple medications, many of which may contribute to constipation. Common culprits are, of course, opioids, but they also include tricyclic antidepressants, anticholinergics, antacids and calcium supplements, iron, diuretics, calcium channel blockers, and antiparkinson drugs.

After addressing reversible causes, clinicians should choose laxatives based on mechanism of action. Senna and bisacodyl act as bowel stimulants. Sorbitol, lactulose, magnesium hydroxide, and polyethylene glycol act by osmotic action to pull water out of the gut lining to effectively flush out stool. Methylcellulose and other bulk-forming agents are not recommended because many patients with terminal illness have diminished fluid intake and run the risk of "cementing" stool in the bowel. Although commonly prescribed, docusate (which acts as a stool softener) has not been shown to be as effective an agent for constipation in more recent studies.[247]

Bisacodyl suppositories stimulate the rectosigmoid colon, whereas glycerin acts as a lubricant and osmotic agent. Enemas (eg, mineral oil, soap suds, or sodium bisphosphate) soften the stool and flush it out. Because rectal insertion is usually unpleasant for patients and caregivers, enemas are only used when other laxatives have proven ineffective or constipation has lasted for more than 5 to 7 days.[248] Administering agents rectally, however, may be indicated and promote the rectal urge to defecate.

The best care involves prevention. Because opioids commonly lead to constipation, clinicians should not only educate the patient and family about this side effect and the importance of aggressive attention to bowel history, but they should also prescribe a standing regimen of laxatives for bowel prophylaxis anytime opioids are ordered. In addition, with increased burden of end-stage disease, decreased activity, and dehydration, the risk of constipation increases. Rather than prescribe bowel regimens based on a specific number of bowel movements per time period, laxative regimens can be adjusted to ensure that patients can have a bowel movement without straining and experiencing incomplete evacuation resulting in cramping abdominal discomfort and gas. In the setting of refractory opioid-induced constipation, newer agents such as methylnaltrexone, a peripheral mu-opioid receptor antagonist, can be used. Studies comparing doses revealed a significant laxation response (approximately 50%, usually within 4 hours) after a 5 mg to 12 mg dose of subcutaneous methylnaltrexone.[249] Dosing recommendations are for a 0.15 mg/kg SC injection (up to 12 mg/dose; reduce by half in severe renal impairment), which is then repeated within 24 to 48 hours if there is no response after the first dose. Side effects include abdominal cramping, flatulence, dizziness, and diarrhea. It does not cause a change in analgesia because the compound does not cross the blood-brain barrier. It is not recommended in the setting of complete bowel obstruction, including severe impaction. Naloxegol, lubiprostone, and oral methylnaltrexone are also FDA approved for opioid-induced constipation and may be considered for patients with constipation refractory to standard laxatives.

Malignant Bowel Obstruction
Prevalence and type of bowel obstruction differ widely given the multiple etiologies and locations of obstruction. Compression of the bowel lumen may develop slowly from either internal or external sources or may be more acute from kinking of the bowel due to mass, adhesions, or malignant ascites. In many cases of malignant obstruction, a combination of medications is helpful: an anticholinergic agent (such as glycopyrrolate) to minimize secretions and colicky pain,[250] a steroid (usually dexamethasone) to decrease peritumor mass effect or bowel edema and inflammation, and a motility agent (eg, metoclopramide) to stimulate peristalsis if bowel obstruction is not complete. If metoclopramide induces more crampy pain, it should be discontinued.

The next step may be a trial of octreotide, a synthetic analog of somatostatin shown to inhibit the release and activity of GI hormones, ultimately decreasing the release of gastric secretions, which slows intestinal motility and reduces splanchnic blood flow.[251] A 2010 multicenter prospective trial demonstrated overall decreased symptoms, and QOL scores improved in 56% of patients treated with octreotide. No serious adverse events were observed.[252] Despite this supportive data, a double-blind, placebo-controlled study calls into question the efficacy of octreotide in malignant bowel obstruction.[253] If prescribed, dosing starts at 100 mcg to 200 mcg SC two to four times a day. If this is not successful, a continuous infusion up to 1,200 mcg daily, or a single dose of a long-acting somatostatin analogue, or a depot somatostatin analogue every 2 to 4 weeks may be administered.[254,255]

The route of drug administration must be individualized. Although a proximal, high-grade obstruction often precludes oral administration, rectal administration is unacceptable to many patients and is problematic when there is a rectal mass, making insertion uncomfortable or even dangerous. SC or IV administration may be preferred, particularly when a central catheter is already in place.

Opioids are used to control associated pain. Additional use of haloperidol orally or subcutaneously is often effective for nausea, but a combination of antiemetics from different classes may be necessary to mitigate refractory nausea. A short trial of IV or SC fluids may be considered to palliate dehydration or thirst if consistent with the patient's goals of care, but evidence of benefit is lacking.[256]

When obstructive symptoms, such as frequent large-volume emesis, persist, the clinician and interdisciplinary team need to clarify goals of care with the patient or decision maker to establish a new plan of care that may include more procedural interventions. **Table 13** outlines pharmacologic treatment options for malignant bowel obstruction.

Table 13. Malignant Bowel Obstruction Treatments

Type of Medication	Dosage
Analgesic	
Morphine sulfate	Titrate upward to efficacy for pain relief
Hydromorphone	Titrate upward to efficacy for pain relief
Anticholinergic	
Scopolamine	1-2 patches (1.5 mg/patch) every 72 hours
Glycopyrrolate	0.8 mg-2 mg a day; can be given in divided dosages or as a continuous infusion[250]
Antidopaminergic	
Haloperidol	0.5 mg-2 mg PO, SL, SC, or IV every 6 hours
Metoclopramide	20 mg-60 mg daily PO, SC, or IV in divided doses every 6 hours or continuous infusion
Other	
Dexamethasone	Loading dose: 4 mg-8 mg PO, SC, or IV Maintenance dose: 4 mg-8 mg twice a day; if no benefit is observed within 5 days, discontinue; if benefit is apparent, after 5 days, begin tapering down until the lowest effective dose is reached
Somatostatin analogues	100 mcg-200 mcg SC or IV three times daily, or up to 1,200 mcg daily as a continuous infusion; long-acting daily or depot formulation administered every 7-28 days

IV, intravenous; PO, by mouth; SC, subcutaneous; SL, sublingual

Procedural Interventions

On some occasions, pharmacologic therapy is either inadequate or inconsistent with patient and family goals or wishes. As a procedural intervention, proximal bowel decompression with an NG tube may serve as a temporizing measure. Sometimes percutaneous venting gastrostomy, self-expanding stents,[257] or surgical bypass with stoma formation can relieve symptoms and improve QOL. These procedures are appropriate to consider for patients with an anticipated life expectancy of at least weeks to months and for whom medical management is not successful. For patients with a good performance status supporting a prognosis of months, and for whom a localized tumor is causing the obstruction, surgical intervention should be considered. Risk factors associated with an increased 30-day mortality include ascites, carcinomatosis, complete small bowel obstruction on imaging,[258] hypoalbuminemia, and abnormal white blood cell count; presence of more of these factors is associated with greater likelihood of death. A review of studies examining the benefits of palliative surgery for malignant bowel obstruction was sobering. Surgery palliated obstructive symptoms for 32% to 100% of patients, enabled resumption of diet for 45% to 75% of patients, and facilitated discharge to home in 34% to 87% of patients.[259] Mortality was high (6%-32%) with median survival of 26 to 237 days. Serious complications were commonplace (7%-44%) and included new obstructions (6%-47%), hospital readmissions (38%-74%), and subsequent operations (2%-15%). Importantly, hospitalization for surgery consumed a substantial portion of the patient's remaining life (11%-61%).[259] Most patients with obstructive symptoms are debilitated with poor performance status, cachexia, significant metastatic disease, and/or ascites so that surgery is not feasible and might be harmful. In such patients, stenting or a venting gastrostomy may provide benefit. Although self-expanding metal stents are less invasive and can be effective,[260,261] other series demonstrate failure or complications in more than 50% of patients treated, including migration, preformation, and occlusion.[262,263]

Delirium

Olga

Olga is an 82-year-old woman with metastatic breast cancer enrolled in hospice home care. She is a widow and lives with her son Bill and daughter-in-law. Bill and his wife plan to travel out of state for their high school reunion and admit Olga to inpatient hospice for respite care for the duration of their 5-day trip.

Olga was enrolled in home hospice 2 months ago on the advice of her oncologist. Recently she has been losing interest in food and has become increasingly weak, spending most of her time in bed. She is still able to swallow and takes duloxetine for depression and oxycodone as needed for her bone pain.

Although Bill is nervous about leaving his mother for a few days, the hospice team assures him she would have visits from volunteers and that they would call immediately with any changes.

During the first 2 days, Olga thrives under the attention of the hospice team. She enjoys visits from hospice volunteers and singing songs with the music therapist. Bill calls daily and is delighted to hear that his mother is doing well, allowing him to enjoy his reunion. On the third day, the day nurse finds Olga more sleepy, and the volunteer is unable to engage her in conversation. She barely eats her breakfast and the nurse notifies the hospice physician. She is asked to name the months of the year backwards, but only names two before she must be reminded to continue the task. She does not have any signs of sensory or motor deficits.

When the hospice on-call nurse arrives, she discovers that Olga has been refusing to take her prescribed oxycodone tablets on a regular schedule for the past 2 days, she has not had a bowel movement for 3 days, and she has been somewhat agitated since the morning. Because of Olga's agitation, the physician prescribes an extra lorazepam tablet twice that day.

Because Olga is suspicious and uncooperative, the physical examination is difficult to perform, but the nurse is able to determine that Olga's pulse is 120, her skin is somewhat dry, her abdomen is mildly distended, and she has a prominent mass in the suprapubic area. Her extremities show muscle wasting and edema, and she will not allow the nurse to check her blood pressure.

? What are known risk factors for delirium?

? How can delirium be prevented or minimized?

? What is the best approach to treating delirium?

Definition and Prevalence

Delirium is a common and distressing phenomenon for patients nearing the end of life and one that remains significantly underdiagnosed by physicians. Studies suggest a prevalence of delirium in 28% to 83% of such patients, depending on the population studied and criteria used.[264] One study of patients in a hospital setting identified an 11% to 42% prevalence of delirium.[265]

Many patients with end-stage illnesses have limited cognitive reserves for a variety of reasons, including but not limited to medication effects, dementia, depression, sleep disturbance, auditory and visual impairment, and dehydration. Other major disease processes known to commonly impair cognitive function include CHF and COPD, both of which can induce hypoxia and/or hypercapnia; HIV/AIDS, which predisposes patients to an array of infections and AIDS-complex dementia; and environmental factors that may further disturb cognitive equilibrium, such as an unfamiliar setting or a lack of day or night cues in an institutional setting.[265]

When an acute brain dysfunction is triggered by one or more factors, as usually is the case, vulnerable patients are much more prone to develop impaired self-orientation and altered consciousness, leading to inattentiveness and impairment in internal and external stimuli perception. See **Table 14** for further characteristics of delirium.

Assessment

The constellation of symptoms needed to diagnose delirium is well defined by a number of measurement tools, including the Confusion Assessment Method (CAM), Delirium Rating Scale, Delirium Symptom Interview, and Memorial Delirium Assessment Scale.[264] The CAM for the intensive care unit (CAM-ICU) has been particularly useful for critically ill patients.[266] Clinicians should remember that delirium can present with hyperactive features (agitation, hallucinations), hypoactive features (lethargy), or features of both types. Differentiating delirium from dementia and depression can be difficult because they share clinical features such as disorientation and impaired thinking and judgment.[267] However, it is important to remember that the onset of delirium is often an acute phenomenon rather than a chronically progressive one, as with dementia. Delirium may be superimposed on underlying dementia,

Table 14. Delirium as Defined by a Constellation of Symptoms[264]

Acute onset

Need to know baseline mental status prior to change, as well as timing and degree of change

Fluctuating course

Waxing/waning in symptoms, usually noted over hours or days

Altered level of consciousness

- Hyperactive, defined by vigilance or agitation
- Hypoactive, defined by lethargy, somnolence, or coma
- Mixed, defined by fluctuation between above states

Inattention

Cognitive impairments

- Altered orientation
- Altered organization of thought; the patient's thinking may be disorganized or incoherent, presenting as rambling or irrelevant conversation, unclear or illogical flow of ideas, or unpredictable switching from subject to subject
- Altered perceptions: delusions or hallucinations, especially visual or auditory
- Emotional lability
- Disruption or reversal of sleep-wake cycle
- Psychomotor agitation or retardation
- Memory impairment

---

particularly for older adults and those with advanced HIV/AIDS. When delirium is suspected, the physician needs to clarify with the patient's surrogate decision maker the desired extent of diagnostic and therapeutic intervention. Before and during this discussion, the provider needs to take into account the degree of distress associated with the delirium, the patient's life expectancy and comorbidities, the location of patient care, and potential burdens of therapies under consideration.

Each of these factors can have a significant influence on a diagnostic evaluation. For example, an aggressive investigation for infectious culprits may be warranted for a patient with end-stage COPD who is still ambulatory. However, if the patient is confused, at home, or at a nursing home, and only expected to live for days, X rays may be too burdensome and not significantly impact the management.

The desired end result of therapy also affects an evaluation. Some patients and families wish to preserve alertness as much as possible to maximize communication. In these cases, a more in-depth diagnostic workup may be appropriate to tailor the therapeutic response. Other patients and families may want to focus on comfort, defined as a degree of sedation to mitigate agitation. In these cases, approximate diagnostic efforts are more limited.

With these goals in mind, the physician will consider the most common and treatable triggers for delirium, performing a focused history and examination to assess for these possibilities. **Table 15** lists some of the more common conditions contributing to delirium by treatability. Bear in mind that most cases of delirium are confounded by a multitude of coexisting medical factors, and many are not reversed with treatment, particularly near the end of life.

Management

General Measures

Management of delirium begins with risk assessment and prevention.[268] As a multifactorial syndrome, delirium is the result of the combination of predisposing conditions and precipitating factors. Patients with higher risk for developing delirium may develop this condition as the result of only a mild condition, whereas patients at much lower risk generally need more severe precipitating factors or a greater number of these factors before delirium occurs. Examples of patients at risk for developing delirium include those with vision impairment, severe illness, cognitive impairment, and dehydration.[269] Precipitants include the use of restraints, increasing polypharmacy, and use of a bladder catheter.

Because this symptom can be dangerous to patients, particularly those with advanced illness, as well as emotionally disturbing to caregivers, it is important to take preventive steps to avoid delirium for every patient receiving palliative care. Providers must consider the impact of every intervention on its likelihood of precipitating delirium and select treatment options least likely to lead to its development. Fortunately delirium can often be prevented with simple environmental changes. Therefore, efforts to educate caregivers (both families and other in-home providers) on recommendations to reduce the incidence are crucial.[270]

The first step is to perform a risk assessment, which can then help guide preventive strategies. Guidelines such as those from the National Institute for Health and Care Excellence (NICE) provide detailed recommendations for prevention.[271,272] Nonpharmacologic interventions that may prevent the onset of delirium include[269,273]

- dehydration prevention
- reorientation and cognitive stimulation
- vision and hearing assessment
- removal of unnecessary catheters, IVs, and restraints
- encouraging appropriate sleep-wake cycles by planning activities during the day, facilitating sunlight exposure, reducing light and sound at night, and minimizing interventions
- induction of sleep with music or massage
- art therapy, aromatherapy
- clarification of concerns or problems, looking specifically for psychosocial or spiritual concerns that may need to be addressed
- education and relaxation techniques

Table 15. Contributing Factors to Delirium

Treatable

Medications such as

- anticholinergics (scopolamine, diphenhydramine, ipratropium)
- opioids or nonsteroidal antiinflammatory drugs
- sedatives, dopamine agonists such as bromocriptine, levodopa, and pergolide
- corticosteroids or antidepressants
- Antibiotics such as fluoroquinolones and sulfonamides
- Cardiovascular agents such as clonidine, digoxin, or beta-blockers
- Gastrointestinal drugs such as H_2 blockers and metoclopramide
- Baclofen or anticonvulsants such as carbamazepine or valproate

Abruptly stopping cardiovascular and centrally acting medications (eg, benzodiazepines, opiates, SSRIs, barbiturates, beta-blockers)

Infections such as

- urinary tract infection
- pneumonia
- any opportunistic infection in immunocompromised patients (eg, HIV/AIDS)

Constipation or urinary retention

Uncontrolled pain

Electrolyte disturbances such as

- hyponatremia or hypernatremia
- hypercalcemia from bone metastases
- hypoglycemia or hyperglycemia

Anemia from blood loss, causing hypoxemia

Dehydration

Immobilization

Depression and social isolation

Vision or hearing impairment

Emotional distress

Unfamiliar environment

Less Treatable

Organ dysfunction at end stages such as

- cardiac or pulmonary failure with ischemia, hypoxia, or hypercapnia
- renal failure
- hepatic failure with encephalopathy
- neurologic dysfunction due to brain metastases, seizure activity, or stroke.

SSRI, selective serotonin reuptake inhibitor.

- change of environment, either bringing in familiar objects to help relieve anxiety or considering admission to a palliative care unit if the home environment or caretakers create added stress for the patient.

Workup

Evaluation of a patient with delirium should include a thorough history and physical exam with special attention to the contributing factors listed in Table 15. All medications, especially those recently changed, should be reviewed. Further investigations should be targeted to address those potentially reversible causes identified in the history and physical exam and carefully aligned with the patient's goals of care. Investigations that can often target easily reversible causes include checking oxygen saturation, testing blood chemistries and blood counts, and looking for infection with urine or blood cultures or a chest X ray.

Treating Reversible Causes

As described in Table 15, many of the causes of delirium are reversible and can be treated if in accordance with the patient's and family's goals of care:

- Opioid toxicity: decrease the dose or rotate to another opioid (usually with less toxic metabolites such as methadone, fentanyl, or hydromorphone).
- Common contributing medications: stop, wean, or decrease possible offending drugs such as benzodiazepines or anticholinergics.
- Infection: start antibiotics considering the goals of care, and remove the nidus of infection, such as an indwelling Foley catheter or central venous line when feasible.
- Dehydration: provide a trial of 500 mL to 1,000 mL of normal saline at a low rate intravenously if it is already present, or infuse subcutaneously; it is important to reassess to ensure therapy is effective and does not cause other side effects such as fluid retention.
- Constipation: see Bowel Obstruction on page 55.
- Urinary retention, hypercalcemia: see Hypercalcemia in the Emergent Conditions chapter on page 77.
- Hypoxia: treat the underlying cause and administer oxygen.

Pharmacologic Management

Given the distressing nature of hyperactive delirium, clinicians often need to start a psychotropic regimen for symptom relief at the same time as the diagnostic evaluation; this gives the clinician time to identify the possible contributors and initiate more focused therapy, such as oral antibiotics for a urinary tract infection. Psychotropic treatment for hypoactive delirium is more controversial. Although some argue that treatment is necessary to reduce the distress caused by this condition, it is unclear whether the benefits outweigh the risks of treatment in this population. Nevertheless, more studies are needed to assess the efficacy of pharmacologic therapy in hypoactive delirium and whether specific agents should be recommended for this subtype. Assistance from a clinical pharmacist can be beneficial.[274] Even when the precipitating cause is treated, however, delirium can persist for weeks to months, or may never completely resolve, and leads to higher rates of nursing home placement, the development of dementia, and increased mortality for affected patients.[275-277]

When using psychotropic medications, the clinician needs to document the specific behavior or behaviors that she is trying to modify to assess the efficacy of therapy and the timing of upward titration, when appropriate. The clinician must also watch for potential side effects of therapy, including insomnia, anorexia, and the precipitation of hyperactive delirium. **Table 16** lists some of the most commonly used psychotropic medications. The goal of therapy is to reduce distress and, if possible, bring the patient back toward their baseline level of mental function. When life expectancy is anticipated to be at least several weeks, it may be appropriate to consider an atypical antipsychotic[278,279] or low-dose haloperidol[280] to minimize the risk of extrapyramidal adverse effects. In addition, when agitation is a prominent feature of delirium that has not responded to a number of agents, it also is appropriate, despite the lack of evidence,[281] to consider the use of a benzodiazepine to cause sedation. This shorter-acting agent offers the advantage of rapid titration; however, each case of delirium needs to be treated on an individual basis, and physicians must carefully assess which psychotropic medication (or combination of medications) is most appropriate.

The uncertainty surrounding psychotropic drugs and delirium in a palliative care population was heightened when a randomized, controlled trial conducted with persons with mild to moderate delirium found no benefit from a low dose of risperidone or haloperidol compared with placebo.[282] The population was predominately patients with cancer, and the outcomes reported were overall differences on a continuous delirium scale of 0.48 and 0.24 units, respectively, compared with placebo. Unfortunately, the authors did not report the more clinically meaningful outcome, which was the proportion of patients with a clinical improvement as defined in the power calculation of a one-point difference on the delirium scale. Moreover, the authors did not report the number of contributors to delirium that were identified and treated or nonpharmacologic interventions implemented because differences in these variables may have contributed to the observed findings. Additional concerns were raised that psychotropics might be associated with increased mortality, which has been demonstrated with older adults with dementia.

Delirium management begins with prevention followed by the treatment of underlying contributors. If the patient's safety is at risk or the patient is suffering as a result of delirium symptoms, pharmacologic treatment should be considered with psychotropics while recognizing the data are, at best, limited.

Black Box Warnings for Antipsychotic Medications
Conventional or atypical antipsychotic medications are not approved to treat dementia-related psychosis because they may cause increased mortality risk for older dementia patients. Most deaths are due to cardiovascular or infectious events; the extent to which increased mortality can be attributed to antipsychotic versus other patient characteristics is not clear.

Table 16. Common Psychotropics for Distress in Delirium

Drug	Indications	Dosing	Contraindications	Adverse Effects
Haloperidol	Most commonly used medication; can use for both hyperactive and hypoactive delirium; titrate for rapid response	0.5 mg-1 mg PO/SL/SC/IV every 2-4 hours or by continuous infusion for acute agitation; titrate to effect for dosing and frequency, up to hourly as needed	Parkinson's disease; will worsen motor symptoms (use quetiapine instead)	Initial worsening of agitation, drug-induced parkinsonian symptoms, dystonia, and prolongation of QTc interval
Risperidone	Less risk for extrapyramidal symptoms, so risperidone is better for long-term use (when life expectancy is weeks to months or longer)	0.25 mg-0.5 mg up to two or three times per day, titrating to relief up to 6 mg per day	Parkinson's disease	Extrapyramidal symptoms, hypotension, paradoxical insomnia, headache Extrapyramidal symptoms increase substantially after 2mg/day
Olanzapine	Less risk for extrapyramidal symptoms; good for long-term use, with side effect profile useful for promoting weight gain	1.25 mg-5 mg once a day, available in wafer form	Parkinson's disease and seizures (lowers seizure threshold)	Sedation, orthostatic hypotension, hyperglycemia, seizures (rare)
Aripiprazole	Negligible effect on QTc, minimally sedating, may be more effective in hypoactive delirium.	5 mg-20 mg once a day	Use with caution in patients with a history of Parkinson's disease or seizures	Sedation, extrapyramidal symptoms, headache, weight gain

Table 16. Common Psychotropics for Distress in Delirium *(continued)*

Drug	Indications	Dosing	Contraindications	Adverse Effects
Quetiapine	Parkinson's-related hallucinations; can use for sedation, particularly at night	12.5 mg–200 mg per day in a single dose or divided doses	Hypotensive states (may potentiate hypertensive medications), seizures (lowers seizure threshold), cataract formation	Sedation, orthostatic hypotension, headaches, dizziness
Valproic Acid	Mood and behavior fluctuations, such as episodic sexually aggressive behavior (evidence weak for agitation in dementia)	125 mg–250 mg every 12 hours, titrating upward to efficacy, with a maximum of 1,000 mg daily in divided dosages	Hepatic dysfunction, including urea-cycle disorders	Primarily GI and neurocognitive disorders such as dyspepsia, nausea and vomiting, diarrhea, somnolence, tremor, headache, and thrombocytopenia
Lorazepam*	Alcohol and substance withdrawal; adjunct for agitated delirium (short-term or actively dying)	0.5 mg–1 mg PO/SL/IV, usually two to four times a day, but can be administered more frequently, up to hourly as needed	Depression, psychosis, central nervous system depressives	Can cause paradoxical agitation, sedation, and transient amnesia

GI, gastrointestinal; IV, intravenous; PO, by mouth; SC, subcutaneous; SL, sublingual.

Usually administered in conjunction with an antipsychotic medication in alternating doses to manage significant agitation that is part of a constellation of delirium symptomatology.

Although multiple trials have shown the benefit of atypical antipsychotics for treating psychosis and behavioral disturbances, their decreased risk for extrapyramidal and movement disorder side effects due to mechanisms of both antidopaminergic and antiserotonergic receptors made them popular choices for patients with dementia when they came into use in the 1990s.[283] The FDA issued a 2005 advisory noting increased mortality among older patients treated with atypical antipsychotic medications, which prompted a good deal of research in the area. A large study compared the risk of death between conventional and atypical antipsychotics; although this study confirmed previous findings of increased mortality with atypical antipsychotics, it raised concern that conventional antipsychotic medications (when used at doses to address behavioral disturbances) led to similar results.[284]

A review of the literature, including a meta-analysis of multiple randomized, placebo-controlled trials and propensity score matching, led many to conclude that these findings should have a direct effect on clinical practice.[285] The results do not contraindicate the use of antipsychotic drugs in the treatment of patients with dementia who have psychotic symptoms and agitation; instead, they change the risk-benefit analysis such that antipsychotic drugs should be used only when there is an identifiable risk of harm to the patient or others, when the distress caused by the symptoms is significant, or when alternate therapies have failed and symptom relief would be beneficial.[286] As with all symptom management, frequent reassessment is necessary to evaluate whether a medication dosage needs to be increased and if the interval of such dosing is adequate to provide continuous relief of delirium. Dosages and dosing intervals may need to increase to break the cycle of agitated delirium; this may lead to sedation, but the clinician may then titrate downward the dosage or dosing intervals to awaken the patient and still control the delirium.

Occasionally, near the end of life, patients experience refractory delirium and restlessness, sometimes referred to as "terminal delirium," which is associated with signs and symptoms that can be difficult to recognize (see **Table 17**).

The physical causes of delirium and restlessness should be considered and, if appropriate, treated with psychological support. Occasionally a physician may have the opportunity to explore psychosocial and spiritual issues with a patient. Intervention efforts should be coordinated with members of the interdisciplinary team, including counselors, social workers, and chaplains. When fears of being alone contribute to restlessness, the continued presence of calming family members, friends, or hospice volunteers can help alleviate a patient's distress.

When no specific problem can be identified and treated and a patient continues to experience anxiety and restlessness, carefully consider titrated doses of lorazepam, 0.5 mg to 2 mg orally, intravenously, subcutaneously, or sublingually as needed; or diazepam, 5 mg to 20 mg tablets crushed in a gelatin capsule and administered per rectum every 6 to 8 hours (per rectum administration may result in erratic absorption and variable efficacy). Higher-dose haloperidol or chlorpromazine can also be effective.

Table 17. Signs of Terminal Delirium

The constellation of symptoms may include the following:

- skin mottling and cool extremities
- mouth breathing with hyperextended neck
- respiratory pattern changes such as Cheyne-Stokes
- calling out for dead family members or friends
- talking about packing bags, taking a trip, going for a car ride (any reference to preparing for a trip)
- periods of deepening somnolence.

When all of the above measures fail to control severe anxiety and terminal restlessness, consider palliative or therapeutic sedation[287] (see *UNIPAC 6*).

Role of Hydration

Similar to other clinical symptom complexes, the question of whether artificial hydration may prevent or reverse terminal delirium is worth considering, given the significant distress and burden delirium causes for patients and caregivers. When a population of terminally ill patients with cancer admitted to an inpatient palliative care unit was studied, researchers found no benefit in either partial opioid substitution or artificial hydration in preventing or reversing delirium during the last week of life.[288] Although this was a small study, it is helpful to remember that any therapy offered should be closely reevaluated to assess for relief of symptoms versus burden of therapy and discontinued if burden increases (such as worsening fluid overload and pulmonary congestion). Literature reviews in 2011 found no evidence that hydration benefits patients with delirium.[256,289]

Emergent Conditions

Clinicians must maintain a high degree of suspicion when emergent conditions (**Table 18**) arise. These conditions, if they are to be treated, require immediate and aggressive management because of their severe impact on the patient and family's QOL.[290] As always, interventions must be appropriate for the patient's and family's goals of care. The sudden onset of a complication in an otherwise minimally symptomatic patient who is expected to have months of survival might justify an evaluation for a disease-oriented or relatively "high-risk" intervention. However, when a patient is debilitated and has a deteriorating condition and a life expectancy of days, an aggressive comfort-oriented approach may be most prudent. When possible, clinicians need to anticipate the development of these conditions; try to prevent them; and prepare patients, families, and the interdisciplinary team. This section does not address uncontrolled pain and delirium, which also require a rapid and thorough response. Those conditions are discussed in *UNIPAC 3* and previously in this book, respectively.

Airway Obstruction

Head and neck tumors, lung cancer, and lymphomas are associated with risk of upper-airway obstruction, which can lead to profound dyspnea and agitation.[291] Prognosis tends to be worse when the trachea or mainstem bronchus is involved or additional antitumor therapy is not warranted.[292] The interdisciplinary team needs to anticipate this complication long before it occurs to discuss goals of care with the patient and family and to implement an agreed-upon treatment plan.[293] For example, has the patient been considered for a mechanical or thermic endoscopic procedure such as rotating microdebridement via bronchoscopy or a radiotherapy ablation technique such as photodynamic therapy, high-dose endobronchial radiotherapy, or brachytherapy?[294-299] If these are not desired, the team may wish to investigate the feasibility of a tracheostomy or bronchial stent.[300]

Opioids and sedatives can effectively palliate the symptoms of dyspnea, air hunger, and anxiety but may cause sedation. This is an effect the patient and family need to anticipate. Some patients want to be alert and comfortable until their final breath, but this may not always be possible. Open discussion and education can defuse conflict and cultivate realistic expectations.

The team also needs to clarify the patient's and family's desired location of care. If and when airway obstruction occurs, do they want death to occur in the home setting or in an inpatient setting? Inpatient care may lead to more rapid and effective symptom management, given the availability of parenteral administration by around-the-clock nursing staff with frequent reassessment. However, continuous or crisis care as mandated by the Medicare hospice benefit may allow for effective management at home as long as the interdisciplinary team is able to plan ahead and address logistical and staffing issues.

Table 18. Common Emergent Conditions

Condition	Common Causes	Symptoms	Possible Treatment
Airway obstruction	Head and neck tumor, lymphoma	Dyspnea, agitation	Bronchoscopic rotating microdebridement, photodynamic therapy, endobronchial radiotherapy or brachytherapy Opioids, benzodiazepines, barbiturates
Cardiac tamponade	Tumor in pericardium, infection, drugs, connective tissue disorder	Dyspnea, cough, orthopnea, dizziness	Pericardiocentesis, indwelling pericardial catheter, percutaneous pericardiostomy, intrapericardial antineoplastic and sclerosing agents
Massive hemorrhage	Tumor evasion into blood vessel	Dyspnea, anxiety	Endovascular procedures, hemostatic dressings, aminocaproic acid, aerosolized vasopressin
Hypercalcemia	Increased PTH/PTHrP secretion, bone metastases	Constipation, fatigue, nausea, bone pain, kidney stones, confusion	Hydration, loop diuretics, bisphosphonates Calcitonin
Pathologic fractures	Bone tumors, osteoporosis	Pain, reduced mobility	Bisphosphonates, denosumab Surgical stabilization Analgesia
Spinal cord compression	Breast, prostate, and lung cancers	Pain, paraparesis, paralysis, incontinence	Steroids, radiotherapy Surgery Gabapentin, pregabalin, tricyclic antidepressants
Seizures	Tumor in CNS	Mental status changes, partial or generalized tonic-clonic movements, incontinence	Benzodiazepines, hydantoins, barbiturates (see Table 20)
Superior vena cava syndrome	Tumor in upper mediastinum	Cough, hoarseness, dyspnea, headache	Steroids Endovascular stenting
Urinary retention	Medications, urethral stricture, lower abdominal tumors, fecal impaction	Oliguria or anuria, restlessness, delirium, abdominal pain	Catheterization (intraurethral, suprapubic) Monitor for postobstructive diuresis

CNS, central nervous system; PTH, parathyroid hormone; PTHrP, parathyroid hormone-related protein

The team needs to have an emergency supply of appropriate medications available in the patient's residence, especially in the setting of a disease that can cause airway obstruction. If medications such as an opioid for dyspnea and a benzodiazepine for anxiety are available before a catastrophic event, the team can teach the family or caregivers how to administer medications appropriately, reinforce the plan that has been decided upon, and reduce the likelihood of a panicked call.

Formulations that have proven useful for airway obstruction include morphine sulfate, 20 mg/mL solution; lorazepam, 2 mg/mL solution; midazolam administered subcutaneously; and phenobarbital administered subcutaneously or compounded as a suppository to be given as needed for anxiety and agitation. The subcutaneous and suppository formulations are helpful when a patient has difficulty handling even minimal volumes of fluids.

If and when the team plans for continuous care in the home or inpatient unit, it may administer continuous parenteral administration of an opioid plus a benzodiazepine such as morphine and lorazepam or midazolam every hour, adjusting every 10 to 15 minutes to reach efficacy. See *UNIPAC 6* for more information about palliative sedation.

Cardiac Tamponade

Cardiac tamponade may result from direct extension or metastatic spread of an underlying malignancy, usually by cancers of the lung and breast, lymphomas, or leukemias.[301] Viral, fungal, and bacterial infections; drugs; connective-tissue disorders; uremia; or a complication of radiation therapy or chemotherapeutic toxicity also can cause this syndrome.[302] Symptoms generally include dyspnea, cough, orthopnea, and dizziness. An examination usually will reveal the classic Beck's triad: hypotension, elevated jugular venous pressure, and distant muffled heart sounds accompanied with tachycardia and pulsus paradoxus. A chest radiograph will often reveal new cardiomegaly, and an electrocardiogram can show low-voltage or electrical alternans.[303] An echocardiogram often reveals a circumferential effusion with collapse of the right atrium and/or ventricle.[304]

Pericardiocentesis provides rapid relief,[305] but malignant pericardial effusions frequently recur. Therapeutic possibilities include an extended indwelling pericardial catheter, percutaneous pericardiostomy, and intrapericardial instillation of antineoplastic and sclerosing agents.[306] Usual treatment involves the surgical creation of a pericardial window that allows the effusion to drain into the pleural space, preventing recurrence of cardiac tamponade.[307] An attractive alternative for debilitated patients, especially if their overall prognosis from the malignancy is poor, is the percutaneous creation of a pericardial window by balloon dilation.[308] If conservative management is desired or the patient is close to death, treatment should focus on symptom control with opioids, benzodiazepines, and oxygen to decrease dyspnea and anxiety.

Massive Hemorrhage

Hemorrhage may occur any time a malignancy erodes into an adjacent blood vessel, leading to catastrophic exsanguination. Head and neck tumors can infiltrate large blood vessels in the neck.[309] Esophageal cancers can grow into major mediastinal vessels. GI tumors can invade mesenteric vessels. Breast cancer can involve subclavian vessels, and pelvic tumors can erode femoral vessels.

Many chronic illnesses and their treatments predispose patients to hemorrhagic risk secondary to thrombocytopenia or clotting dysfunction. This is commonly seen in cancers that infiltrate the bone marrow after myeloablative chemotherapies and in coagulopathy related to liver failure. This risk is further complicated by medications that limit coagulation (aspirin, warfarin, Xa inhibitor [lepirudin or argatroban], nonsteroidal antiinflammatory drugs [NSAIDs]) or is related to acute infection and subsequent disseminated intravascular coagulation.

The interdisciplinary team needs to think critically about the complications of a patient's diagnosis and anticipate the progression and severity of a potential hemorrhagic event. As with all other symptoms, adequate preemptive discussions and planning regarding the desired goals of care lead to provision of agreed-upon treatment and avoidance of unwanted emergency interventions. A careful review of the cause of bleeding risks may reveal treatable factors.[310,311]

Aspirin, other NSAIDs, and anticoagulants such as warfarin and Xa inhibitors should be discontinued when hemorrhage is a concern. The burden-to-benefit ratio of other medications such as steroids may need to be reconsidered. In addition, the patient may be a candidate for interventional procedures such as banding, sclerotherapy, radiotherapy, or vascular embolization, which may limit or prevent acute bleeding episodes.

To control anticipated or recurrent bleeding for which compression is not effective, consider endovascular procedures,[309,312] hemostatic dressings for surface wounds,[313] aminocaproic acid for bleeding for patients with thrombocytopenia,[314] or aerosolized vasopressin for hemoptysis.[315] Other systemic treatment considerations that might be considered depending upon goals of care include plasma products, platelets when less than 10,000 to 20,0000, vitamin K, and vasopressin. Prothrombin complex concentrate has been used to reverse anticoagulation that occurs with Xa inhibitors and others, but its high cost limits its use, particularly in hospice.[316] Opioids should be used to treat pain or respiratory distress, and sedatives should be used to relieve anxiety. The team should inform the family and caregivers that a massive arterial bleed is painless and death can occur quickly. If a hemorrhage is perceived to be a real possibility, the patient's bed should be made up with dark sheets and blankets, and quantities of dark towels should be kept at the bedside to absorb and mask the blood. Even if death is rapid and painless, what family members will always retain is the visual memory of red blood against white linens; it is a kindness to them to prevent this memory, if possible.

Hypercalcemia

Hypercalcemia will occur in 20% to 30% of all patients with cancer and is most commonly seen in non-small cell lung cancer, breast cancer, head and neck cancer, renal-cell cancer, multiple myeloma, and T-cell lymphoma.[317] Eighty percent of all cases of hypercalcemia are caused by the parathyroid hormone-like peptide that is produced by a variety of malignancies. In addition, direct bony destruction from cytokines from metastases also leads to hypercalcemia.[318] Direct calcitriol production occurs infrequently for some patients with Hodgkin disease. Symptomatic hypercalcemia can be remembered by the mnemonic presented in **Table 19**.[319]

Serum calcium binds to albumin, and a hypoalbuminemia, which is often present for patients with advanced malignancies, will lead to a falsely decreased calcium reading. Consequently, an approximate correction factor should be used: for every 1 g decrement of albumin below the baseline of 4.0 g, add 0.8 mg of calcium. (For example, if a patient has an albumin level of 2.5 g and reported serum calcium of 8.0 mg/dL, the corrected calcium level is 9.2 mg/dL.)

Intervention needs to be appropriate to reflect the patient's wishes, overall status, and the underlying malignancy. In debilitated patients with hypercalcemia from a malignancy that does not respond to treatment, survival usually is only a few weeks. It may be decided that optimal intervention is to withhold hypercalcemia treatment. If the prognosis is judged to be longer and the patient and family want interventions, they should consist primarily of volume expansion to increase filtered load of calcium, loop diuretics (after adequate hydration) to inhibit resorption of calcium in the loop of Henle, and bisphosphonate treatment.[320] Also important is a thorough medication review to eliminate extraneous sources of calcium (calcium in total parenteral nutrition; supplements including calcium, vitamin D and antacids; lithium and thiazides). Calcitonin is another modality for acute treatment (dose 4 units/kg SC/IM every 12 hours, up to 8 units/kg every 6 hours) but is not commonly used because its effects are only transient and side effects include tachyphylaxis.[321,322] Denosumab, a fully human monoclonal antibody, is now FDA approved for malignancy-related hypercalcemia refractory to bisphosphonates.[323]

Bisphosphonates are now the mainstay for therapy; options include pamidronate, 60 mg to 90 mg diluted in 500 mL to 1,000 mL of normal saline administered intravenously (but not subcutaneously) over 4 to 6 hours; or zoledronate, 4 mg administered intravenously over at least 15 minutes. Effect should be seen after 2 to 4 days, and doses can be repeated after 1 to 3 weeks as needed, exercising care to watch for hypocalcemia, hypophosphatemia, and hypomagnesemia. An important adverse effect of prolonged therapy is the risk of osteonecrosis of the jaw (ONJ), which is thought to be secondary to the strong inhibition of osteoclast function precipitated by bisphosphonate therapy, leading to inhibition of normal bone turnover.[324] According to a 2014 medication-related osteonecrosis of the jaw position paper published by the American Association of Oral and Maxillofacial Surgeons, the potency of and length of exposure to bisphosphonates are linked to risk for developing bisphosphonate-related

Table 19. Symptomatic Hypercalcemia[319]

Groans	Constipation
Moans	Fatigue, lethargy, nausea
Bones	Bone pain
Stones	Kidney stones
Psychiatric overtones	Including depression and confusion

osteonecrosis of the jaw.[325] Studies have estimated occurrence in up to 20% of patients taking zoledronic acid intravenously for cancer therapy and between 0% to 0.04% of patients taking orally administered bisphosphonates.[326] Prevention is key. The Canadian Association of Oral and Maxillofacial Surgeons consensus guidelines recommend the following:

In all oncology patients, a thorough dental examination including radiographs should be completed prior to the initiation of intravenous bisphosphonate therapy. In this population, any invasive dental procedure is ideally completed prior to the initiation of high-dose bisphosphonate therapy. Non-urgent procedures are preferably delayed for 3 to 6 months following interruption of bisphosphonate therapy. Osteoporosis patients receiving oral or intravenous bisphosphonates do not require a dental examination prior to initiating therapy in the presence of appropriate dental care and good oral hygiene. Stopping smoking, limiting alcohol intake, and maintaining good oral hygiene should be emphasized for all patients receiving bisphosphonate therapy. Individuals with established ONJ are most appropriately managed with supportive care including pain control, treatment of secondary infection, removal of necrotic debris, and mobile sequestrate. Aggressive debridement is contraindicated.[327]

Pathologic Fractures

Within the palliative care population there are many risk factors that predispose patients to pathologic fractures, including osteoporosis, primary bone tumors, and metastatic disease. The goals are first to identify at-risk groups to prevent fractures and then, if present, to tailor their treatment to alleviate pain, restore function, and prevent neurologic sequelae.

Regardless of etiology, any process that weakens bony structure can elicit pain, often preceding pathologic fracture. In an effort to provide preventive measures, appropriate screening for at-risk patients is key to improving overall morbidity and mortality, including subsequent fractures. Of course, treatment of underlying disease (whether osteoporosis or a malignant cancer) is optimal, but if it is not possible to cure underlying disease, treatment should focus on inhibition of bone resorption with bisphosphonates.

Although bisphosphonates have not been shown to be beneficial in managing large, lytic metastases, they are certainly useful in osteoporotic disease and for smaller, more diffuse metastatic disease.[328] Many studies confirm that the use of regular bisphosphonates (monthly pamidronate IV or zoledronic acid) can help relieve pain and decrease the rate of skeletal complications.[329] No clear association between bisphosphonates and fractures of the femur has been found, and these rarely occur.[330-332] Denosumab appears to be effective for reducing skeletal events for patients with metastatic prostate cancer[333] or breast cancer and may increase bone metastasis–free survival.[334]

In addition to optimizing conservative medical therapies, orthopedic intervention can be important when impending or pathologic fracture or spinal instability are present. For the vast majority of patients, internal stabilization or replacement arthroplasty are the best alternatives, but type and specifics are dependent on location and extensiveness of disease, with an ultimate goal to restore unsupported use of the limb.[328] Innovative percutaneous fixation methods that effectively relieve pain are being refined,[335,336] so consultation with an oncologic orthopedist may be fruitful.

Surgical stabilization often requires extensive surgeries; effort has been made to investigate less invasive procedures. For example, vertebroplasty and kyphoplasty are less complicated day-surgery approaches to stabilizing spinal compression fractures. Initial trials of these approaches showed good evidence for superior pain control and fair evidence for less analgesic use and better return to function over more conservative medical management.[337] However, other studies comparing vertebroplasty procedures to control groups using sham procedures revealed no significant advantage in any measured outcomes, specifically pain, physical functioning, and QOL.[338,339] Pain improved modestly in both groups over time, perhaps pointing to previous studies' overestimates of treatment benefit by failing to take into account the natural healing of compression fractures and the placebo response to treatment.[338,339] Despite these revelations, the use of kyphoplasty, in particular, continues to grow.[340]

Contraindications to surgery include terminal illness with a prognosis shorter than 2 to 4 weeks, high risk for surgical stabilization failure secondary to extensive bony destruction, and presence of infection. Models are being developed that appear to predict with some accuracy the time at which a pathological fracture is most likely to occur in some circumstances.[341] Unfortunately, perhaps because of overemphasis on contraindications or lack of education among physicians, many candidates are not referred for surgical intervention to treat pathologic fracture and/or prevent worsening decompensation of bony disease.[328]

Surgery alone is often inadequate, necessitating interdisciplinary management to include physical and rehabilitative therapies, nutrition, wound management, postoperative radiotherapy, continued or supplemental treatment of tumor with hormone therapy or chemotherapy, and medical stabilization of bone with bisphosphonates. For more information about the treatment of bone pain, see *UNIPAC 3*.

Spinal Cord Compression

Approximately 2.5% of patients with cancer will have spinal cord compression at the end of their lives, putting them at risk for pain, paraparesis or paralysis, incontinence, and hospitalization.[342] This condition most commonly is seen in breast, prostate, and lung cancers (each accounting for 15%-20% of cases), followed by lymphomas, myeloma, and renal-cell cancer (each with 10%-15% of cases). The remainder of patients primarily have colorectal cancer, cancer of unknown primary, and sarcomas.[343,344] Epidural and locally advanced metastasis make up the majority of spinal cord compression cases, with approximately 90% originating from vertebral metastasis and 10% being foraminal. The interdisciplinary team needs to consider the possibility of vertebral or epidural spine metastases for any patient with malignancy and new back pain because 83% to 95% experience back pain prior to the diagnosis.[345] Look for central back pain aggravated by movement or Valsalva-like activities (eg, coughing, sneezing, or straining while having a bowel movement), radicular pain wrapping around the rib cage or down one or both legs, urinary retention with overflow incontinence, fecal incontinence, or progressive distal motor or sensory polyneuropathy.

Recognizing symptoms of spinal cord compression is crucial because a delay in diagnosis can result in loss of mobility, bladder dysfunction, and decreased survival.[346] Moreover, the ability to ambulate prior to treatment is a significant predictor of preserved ambulation after treatment. Although the cause of damage to the spinal cord is complex, two mechanisms predominate: direct compression resulting in edema, venous congestion, and demyelination (typically reversible) and prolonged compression, resulting in infarction of the spinal cord (irreversible).[347] If radiation or surgery is being considered, early diagnosis and treatment within 24 to 48 hours of an impending cord compression is critical to preserve neurologic function. Magnetic resonance imaging (MRI) of the entire spine is the gold standard, because about one-third of cord compressions have multiple metastatic sites that can often change the course of treatment.[348]

Standard treatment for metastatic epidural spinal cord compression consists of corticosteroids and radiotherapy.[349,350] The role of corticosteroids (typically dexamethasone) is to inhibit the inflammatory cascade, decreasing vasogenic edema and subsequent tissue damage. Historically, debate existed between using high-dose dexamethasone (100 mg loading, then 96 mg daily) versus a more moderate dose (10 mg loading, then 16 mg daily). A randomized, controlled trial comparing the two doses found no differences in efficacy; thus, most clinicians give the lower dose. Many studies give the steroids divided four times a day, tapered over 10 to 14 days. The steroid generally is administered intravenously to start then switched to oral administration when patients are "clinically stable" and more definitive therapy (radiation or surgery) has been initiated. Steroids should be tapered as soon as possible to prevent long-term toxicities.

Radiation therapy is directed at vertebral metastases that are painful or are associated with significant spinal cord involvement. Standard therapy usually consists of 10 fractions; however, courses may be prolonged (up to 25 fractions) or shortened based on life expectancy.[348] For patients with a poor prognosis, a single fraction of 8 Gy is just as effective as multiple fractions and much more convenient.[351]

Debate is ongoing regarding the merits of radiotherapy alone versus surgical therapy followed by radiation for selected patients. Standard therapy results in 50% of patients with metastatic epidural spinal cord compression being able to walk after radiation alone.[347] An updated 2011 evidence-based review recommended radiation for all patients not undergoing primary surgery and without spinal instability, bony compression, or paraplegia on presentation; it recommended surgical decompression for patients with progressive neurologic deficits, vertebral column instability, radio-resistant tumors (lung, colon, renal cell), and intractable pain unrelieved by radiation therapy.[351] The first published prospective, randomized trial comparing the efficacy of direct decompressive surgery followed by radiotherapy versus radiotherapy alone in a group of 100 patients resulted in early discontinuation because of the superior response of the group randomized to surgery. The primary endpoint was the ability to walk after treatment (84% in the surgery group versus 57% with radiation alone), with noted longer maintenance of effects (122 days versus 13 days). Secondary endpoints included urinary continence, changes in functional scores, and decreased use of corticosteroids and opiates.[350] The results of this trial cannot be used to justify surgery in all patients because the patient population studied consisted only of those for whom surgery was a realistic option. However, perhaps the results can be applied to patients comparable to those in the study. Physicians should carefully weigh a patient's ability to tolerate surgery and the goals of care before recommending any significant procedure. Minimally invasive surgical techniques are being developed for palliative care patients.[352]

Regardless of aggressiveness of radiotherapy or surgical decompression, pain and symptom management during this process are integral to adequate treatment. It is not uncommon to initially see a significant escalation in opiate requirements, often necessitating continuous infusion of opioids delivered through a patient-controlled analgesic device. Neuropathic pain adjuvants (eg, gabapentin, pregabalin, tricyclics, serotonin-norepinephrine reuptake inhibitors) have been shown to decrease paresthesias and burning radicular pains associated with peripheral nerve and spinal-cord injury and have an opioid-sparing effect.[353] Similarly, intravenous bisphosphonates have been shown to decrease bone pain with vertebral involvement (for more information, see the Pathologic Fractures on page 78).[284] If patients have widespread bony metastases and a prognosis of months, treatment with a radioisotope (eg, strontium-89) may be a consideration.[354] If nerve damage is severe, aggressive treatment of symptoms such as urinary retention and constipation resulting from autonomic dysfunction is imperative and may require intermittent catheterizations and daily stimulant suppositories.[348]

Seizures

Seizures usually are recognized by acute mental status changes,[355] partial or generalized tonic-clonic movements, or incontinence. Seizures in the palliative care setting occur most often with patients with cerebral or leptomeningeal malignancy and less frequently with patients with metabolic disturbances, infection, drug toxicity, drug withdrawal, and intracerebral hemorrhage.

Although some argue the role of prophylactic antiepileptic medication for patients with advanced brain tumors,[356,357] the American Academy of Neurology's practice parameter (last updated in 2008) does not recommend prophylactic use of these drugs. This is based on a lack of evidence that the therapy will prevent first-time seizures[358] as well as the risk profile, discomfort, expense, and inconvenience of anticonvulsant medications.[359] Workup and treatment of subsequent seizures can become complicated and, as always, should be based on the patient's and family's goals of care. When patients maintain relatively preserved functional status and have longer life expectancies, it may be appropriate to offer diagnostic studies urgently, such as head CT or MRI scan and, when appropriate, further therapy such as radiation and even surgical resection.

Nonconvulsive status epilepticus (NCSE) remains challenging in both diagnosis and treatment but may be a potentially reversible cause of altered mental status or delirium.[360,361] Although data are limited, NCSE has been reported in up to 6% of patients with systemic cancer without evidence of CNS involvement, and in up to 20% of patients with known primary CNS malignancies or metastases.[362] Other studies suggest brain tumors only account for up to 10% of cases of NCSE in older people, with ischemic stroke and intracranial hemorrhage causing up to 40%, hypoxia causing 17%, and metabolic disturbances 14%.[363] Recognizing and managing NCSE is important because studies have shown that early effective treatment can restore communicative abilities, even in severely ill patients.[364]

An antiepileptic medication may be selected based on type of seizure, route of administration, enzyme induction, and accessibility.[365] Diagnosis of primary seizure disorders and subsequent treatment is left in the domain of neurologists; we will focus on management of seizures within the palliative care setting, specifically refractory seizures and status epilepticus.[366] Although certain medications can be administered subcutaneously or rectally when a patient wants to stay at home and does not have intravenous access, the patient and family should understand that sedation is often an anticipated side effect of efforts to control seizures. **Table 20** shows many of the common medications used to treat seizures.

Initial studies and literature review led to the algorithm for the treatment of NCSE involving a stepwise approach. The first tier recommends using benzodiazepines and phenytoin, showing 8% to 24% efficacy; the second recommends replacing phenytoin with valproic acid or a barbiturate, possibly with continued midazolam, increasing efficacy to 63%; third, using levetiracetam (supported only by anecdotal evidence because it is newer to the market; see next paragraph) or lidocaine (1.5 mg/kg to 2 mg/kg IV bolus, followed by 2 mg/kg to 4 mg/kg

Table 20. Seizure Medications for Status Epilepticus in the Palliative Care Setting

Medication	Dosage	Comments
Benzodiazepines		
Lorazepam	0.05 mg/kg-0.1 mg/kg (usually 2 mg-5 mg) IV/SC/SL bolus (may repeat once after 5-10 minutes), followed by 1 mg-2 mg hourly as needed	First-line for isolated seizure activity Not recommended alone for status epilepticus
Midazolam	0.15 mg/kg IV, then 1 mcg/kg/min infusion, titrated to effect May also be administered intranasally as needed for acute seizure control	Best for infusion Quickest onset of action
Diazepam	0.2 mg/kg-0.5 mg/kg (up to 20 mg) PR; may repeat once in 4-12 hours (in home setting) or 0.1 mg/kg-0.3 mg/kg (usually 5 mg-10 mg) IV every 5-10 minutes (max 30 mg)	More sedating Longer duration of action Preset rectal applicators available, specifically for home use
Hydantoins		
Phenytoin	15 mg/kg-20 mg/kg (up to 1 g) IV bolus (give at 50 mg/min, may repeat 5 mg/kg-10 mg/kg once after 20 minutes), then 5 mg/kg-8 mg/kg PO/IV divided twice daily	Drug-level monitoring, adjusted for albumin Decreased plasma levels when given with steroids IV formulation can cause local irritation, damage if it infiltrates
Fosphenytoin	15 mg/kg-20 mg/kg PE IV bolus (150 mg PE/min), then 4 mg/kg-6 mg/kg PE IV/SC daily	Less locally irritating than phenytoin
Barbiturates		
Phenobarbital	20 mg/kg IV bolus (give at 100 mg/min, may repeat 5 mg/kg-10 mg/kg every 15 minutes to max 40 mg/kg), followed by 5 mg/kg-8 mg/kg divided twice daily	More sedating Can cause lower ICP; can be given SC or PR if needed
Other		
Valproic acid	25 mg/kg-45 mg/kg bolus IV at up to 3 mg/kg/min, up to 60 mg/kg/day	Less sedating, less hypotensive side effects Multiple drug interactions Can be given PO or PR
Levetiracetam	1,000 mg-2,000 mg IV, up to 3,000 mg/day	Very few interactions No need for drug levels

ICP, intracranial pressure; IV, intravenous; PE, phenytoin equivalents; PO, by mouth; PR, per rectum; SC, subcutaneous; SL, sublingual.

hourly if needed, increasing efficacy to 74% and 95%, respectively). Overall, goals for patients in palliative settings differ from goals in other settings because patients and families usually want to avoid the use of general anesthesia (such as propofol), which could necessitate intubation and ICU care to manage seizures.[367] The interdisciplinary team can be especially effective under such difficult circumstances.[368]

A subsequent secondary study revealed that a newer agent, levetiracetam, may have better efficacy in the NCSE setting. This study included 15 patients admitted to a palliative care unit with delirium in NCSE; only one patient responded to phenytoin and another to valproic acid. Seven patients, however, responded to levetiracetam, resulting in a total 9 of 15 patients with resolution of NCSE; these patients regained consciousness and the ability to communicate (four of whom presented in comas). Time to response ranged from 4 hours to 6 days, which encouraged longer time trials than previously recommended. Seizures reoccurred in all but one patient, but survival ranged between 11 and 184 days.[364]

Superior Vena Cava Syndrome

Superior vena cava (SVC) syndrome encompasses a constellation of symptoms and signs resulting from obstruction of the SVC, usually occurring with malignant encroachment in the upper-right mediastinum as a result of primary or metastatic lung cancer and lymphomas.[369,370] SVC syndrome also can be associated with thrombosis, a common complication of central venous catheters in the setting of a malignancy-associated hypercoagulable state. Astute clinicians will identify facial plethora, facial and upper-extremity edema, dilated collateral veins over the chest wall, and distention of arm veins that is unrelieved when the patient's arms are elevated.[371] Worsening edema leads to functional compromise and gradual onset of symptoms, including cough and hoarseness from vocal cord edema, headache from cerebral edema, dyspnea, and hemodynamic compromise.[372]

When such a diagnosis is made, the interdisciplinary team needs to stress the importance of elevating the patient's head and avoiding venipunctures and IV access in the upper extremities. Steroids may reduce peritumor edema and partially decompress the SVC syndrome, particularly for patients with lymphoma. One proposed regimen is dexamethasone, 6 mg to 10 mg orally or intravenously two to four times a day. Before the availability of endovascular stenting, catheter-associated SVC syndrome was successfully treated with thrombolytics[373] or tPA.[374] Loop diuretics are commonly used, but evidence is unclear whether venous pressure distal to the obstruction is affected by small changes in right atrial pressure.[372]

When the tumor is chemosensitive, patients may benefit from chemotherapy, particularly patients who are chemotherapy-naïve, have a life expectancy of at least months, and have pronounced symptoms related to SVC syndrome. Studies show complete symptom relief of SVC obstruction with chemotherapy in up to 80% of patients with non-Hodgkin lymphoma or small cell lung cancer, and in 40% of patients with non-small cell lung cancer.[372] When a tumor is not chemosensitive and a patient still has an adequately long prognosis, radiation therapy, surgical and/or imagery guided techniques,[375] or endovascular stenting[376,377] are options. The interdisciplinary team, in consultation with the patient's oncologist, should balance the benefits and burdens of any treatment plan, which includes both diagnostic and therapeutic interventions and their subsequent logistics and costs.

Urinary Retention

A sudden acute decrease in urinary output associated with blockage of urinary flow and retention of urine can be distressing for patients. Symptoms can be slowly progressive, starting as decreased urinary stream, hesitancy, frequency, inability to fully empty the bladder, or incontinence; some presentations are less insidious. Acute lower tract obstruction usually causes extreme discomfort as the bladder becomes overdistended and can be palpated on exam.[378] Depending on the baseline mental status of the patient, acute urinary retention may present instead as restlessness, diaphoresis, or delirium.

Complete cessation of urinary flow usually implies obstruction of the lower urinary tract at the bladder neck, prostate, or urethra, or an upper tract obstruction of either a functioning single kidney or, less frequently, bilateral ureters. Clinicians should do a thorough medication review to look for drugs that may cause urinary retention, such as anticholinergics, alpha-adrenergic medications, or new opioids. In addition, a recent history of urethral manipulation may cause a stricture.[379] Physical exam may reveal a palpable bladder or other abdominal masses or ascites, which could point to etiology of obstruction. A rectal examination is paramount because prostate pathology, rectal masses, or severe impaction can contribute to symptoms of urinary retention.

For lower urinary obstruction, the most appropriate treatment is passing a catheter to drain the bladder; the catheter may be impregnated with silver alloy or an antibiotic to reduce infection risk.[379] If anatomy precludes catheter placement, a suprapubic catheter may be necessary until further diagnostics can be obtained or placed for the long term in some cases.[380] Upper urinary obstruction can be more complicated because the etiology usually is more malignant, secondary to tumor invasion or compression of ureters by retroperitoneal fibrosis or lymphadenopathy. Urologic evaluation for indwelling ureteral stents or percutaneous nephrostomy drainage may be necessary (depending on goals of the patient and family), but evidence of improved QOL or significant survival advantage is lacking.[381] Occasionally pelvic tumors present with urinary obstruction, and courses of chemotherapy, radiation, or hormone blockade can quickly alleviate symptoms while treating the underlying disease process.

It is important to monitor urinary output both before and after relief of obstruction for postobstructive diuresis, which can lead to worsening renal failure. If a patient diureses too quickly, it may become necessary to clamp the catheter to slow diuresis and avoid volume depletion.

Ultimately, if urinary obstruction results from a progressive, incurable pathology, it is worthwhile to discuss all options for treatment and also the possibility of bypassing treatment and focusing on palliative symptom management instead of prolongation of life and potential suffering.[382]

For more detailed information about acute management of emergent conditions, clinicians should refer to other resources, including the articles referenced in this book and textbooks such as the *Oxford Textbook of Palliative Medicine, 5th Edition*.[383] Clinical suspicion, careful examination, and good communication with other team members[384] and the patient and family are essential to manage these urgent conditions.[290] All therapies should do more good than harm and be in accord with the patient's wishes.[385]

References

1. Chang VT, Hwang SS, Feuerman M. Validation of the Edmonton Symptom Assessment Scale. *Cancer.* 2000;88(9):2164-2171.

2. Chang VT, Hwang SS, Feuerman M, Kasimis BS, Thaler HT. The memorial symptom assessment scale short form (MSAS-SF). *Cancer.* 2000;89(5):1162-1171.

3. Murray TM, Sachs GA, Stocking C, Shega JW. The symptom experience of community-dwelling persons with dementia: self and caregiver report and comparison with standardized symptom assessment measures. *Am J Geriatr Psychiatry.* 2012;20(4):298-305.

4. O'Donnell DE, Banzett RB, Carrieri-Kohlman V, et al. Pathophysiology of dyspnea in chronic obstructive pulmonary disease: a roundtable. *Proc Am Thorac Soc.* 2007;4(2):145-168.

5. Nishino T. Dyspnoea: underlying mechanisms and treatment. *Br J Anaesth.* 2011;106(4):463-474.

6. Ripamonti C, Bruera E. Dyspnea: pathophysiology and assessment. *J Pain Symptom Manage.* 1997;13(4):220-232.

7. Claessens MT, Lynn J, Zhong Z, et al. Dying with lung cancer or chronic obstructive pulmonary disease: insights from SUPPORT. Study to Understand Prognoses and Preferences for Outcomes and Risks of Treatments. *J Am Geriatr Soc.* 2000;48(5 Suppl):S146-153.

8. Greenberg B, McCorkle R, Vlahov D, Selwyn PA. Palliative care for HIV disease in the era of highly active antiretroviral therapy. *J Urban Health.* 2000;77(2):150-165.

9. McCarthy M, Lay M, Addington-Hall J. Dying from heart disease. *J R Coll Physicians Lond.* 1996;30(4):325-328.

10. Addington-Hall J, Lay M, Altmann D, McCarthy M. Symptom control, communication with health professionals, and hospital care of stroke patients in the last year of life as reported by surviving family, friends, and officials. *Stroke.* 1995;26(12):2242-2248.

11. Voltz R, Borasio GD. Palliative therapy in the terminal stage of neurological disease. *J Neurol.* 1997;244(Suppl 4):S2-10.

12. Reuben DB, Mor V. Dyspnea in terminally ill cancer patients. *Chest.* 1986;89(2):234-236.

13. Kamal AH, Swetz KM, Liu H, et al. Survival trends in palliative care patients with cancer: a Mayo Clinic 5-year review. *J Clin Oncol.* 2009;27(15S):9592-9592.

14. Barbera L, Taylor C, Dudgeon D. Why do patients with cancer visit the emergency department near the end of life? *CMAJ.* 2010;182(6):563-568.

15. Mercadante S, Casuccio A, Fulfaro F. The course of symptom frequency and intensity in advanced cancer patients followed at home. *J Pain Symptom Manage.* 2000;20(2):104-112.

16. Abernethy AP, Wheeler JL. Total dyspnoea. *Curr Opin Support Palliat Care.* 2008;2(2):110-113.

17. Thomas JR, von Gunten CF. Clinical management of dyspnoea. *Lancet Oncol.* 2002;3(4):223-228.

18. Loring SH, Garcia-Jacques M, Malhotra A. Pulmonary characteristics in COPD and mechanisms of increased work of breathing. *J Appl Physiol.* 2009;107(1):309-314.

19. Nishimura K, Izumi T, Tsukino M, Oga T. Dyspnea is a better predictor of 5-year survival than airway obstruction in patients with COPD. *Chest.* 2002;121(5):1434-1440.

20. Narducci F, Grande R, Mentuccia L, et al. Symptom improvement as prognostic factor for survival in cancer patients undergoing palliative care: a pilot study. *Support Care Cancer.* 2011.

21. Goldberg R, Goff D, Cooper L, et al. Age and sex differences in presentation of symptoms among patients with acute coronary disease: the REACT Trial. Rapid Early Action for Coronary Treatment. *Coron Artery Dis.* 2000;11(5):399-407.

22. McSweeney JC, Cody M, O'Sullivan P, Elberson K, Moser DK, Garvin BJ. Women's early warning symptoms of acute myocardial infarction. *Circulation.* 2003;108(21):2619-2623.

23.   Campbell EJM, Howell JBL. The sensation of dyspnea. *BMJ*. 1963;2:868.

24.   Mioxham J, Jolley C. Breathlessness, fatigue and the respiratory muscles. *Clin Med (Northfield Il)*. 2009;9(5):448-452.

25.   Campbell EJM, Howell JBL. The sensation of breathlessness. *Br Med Bull*. 1963;19:36-40.

26.   Kamal AH, Maguire JM, Wheeler JL, Currow DC, Abernethy AP. Dyspnea review for the palliative care professional: assessment, burdens, and etiologies. *J Palliat Med*. 2011;14(10):1167-1172.

27.   Moy ML, Reilly JJ, Ries AL, et al. Multivariate models of determinants of health-related quality of life in severe chronic obstructive pulmonary disease. *J Rehabil Res Dev*. 2009;46(5):643-654.

28.   Reddy SK, Parsons HA, Elsayem A, Palmer JL, Bruera E. Characteristics and correlates of dyspnea in patients with advanced cancer. *J Palliat Med*. 2009;12(1):29-36.

29.   Campbell ML. Dyspnea. *AACN Adv Crit Care*. 2011;22(3):257-264.

30.   Tanaka K, Akechi T, Okuyama T, Nishiwaki Y, Uchitomi Y. Development and validation of the Cancer Dyspnoea Scale: a multidimensional, brief, self-rating scale. *Br J Cancer*. 2000;82(4):800-805.

31.   Wysham NG, Miriovsky BJ, Currow DC, et al. Practical dyspnea assessment: relationship between the 0-10 numerical rating scale and the four-level categorical verbal descriptor scale of dyspnea intensity. *J Pain Symptom Manage*. 2015;50(4):480-487.

32.   Campbell ML, Templin T, Walch J. A Respiratory Distress Observation Scale for patients unable to self-report dyspnea. *J Palliat Med*. 2010;13(3):285-290.

33.   Persichini R, Gay F, Schmidt M, et al. Diagnostic accuracy of respiratory distress observation scales as surrogates of dyspnea self-report in intensive care unit patients. *Anesthesiology*. 2015;123(4):830-837.

34.   Davies HE, Mishra EK, Kahan BC, et al. Effect of an indwelling pleural catheter vs chest tube and talc pleurodesis for relieving dyspnea in patients with malignant pleural effusion: the TIME2 randomized controlled trial. *JAMA*. 2012;307(22):2383-2389.

35.   Corner J, Plant H, A'Hern R, Bailey C. Non-pharmacological intervention for breathlessness in lung cancer. *Palliat Med*. 1996;10(4):299-305.

36.   Marciniuk D, Goodridge D, Hernandez P, et al. Managing dyspnea in patients with advanced chronic obstructive pulmonary disease: a Canadian Thoracic Society clinical practice guideline. *Can Respir J*. 2011;18(2):69-78.

37.   Galbraith S, Fagan P, Perkins P, Lynch A, Booth S. Does the use of a handheld fan improve chronic dyspnea? A randomized, controlled, crossover trial. *J Pain Symptom Manage*. 2010;39(5):831-838.

38.   Kemp C. Palliative care for respiratory problems in terminal illness. *Am J Hosp Palliat Care*. 1997;14(1):26-30.

39.   Kelly CA, O'Brien MR. Difficult decisions: an interpretative phenomenological analysis study of healthcare professionals' perceptions of oxygen therapy in palliative care. *Palliat Med*. 2015;29(10):950-958.

40.   Nocturnal Oxygen Therapy Trial Group. Continuous or nocturnal oxygen therapy in hypoxemic chronic obstructive lung disease: a clinical trial. *Ann Intern Med*. 1980;93(3):391-398.

41.   Long term domiciliary oxygen therapy in chronic hypoxic cor pulmonale complicating chronic bronchitis and emphysema. Report of the Medical Research Council Working Party. *Lancet*. 1981;317(8222):681-686.

42.   Eaton T, Lewis C, Young P, Kennedy Y, Garrett JE, Kolbe J. Long-term oxygen therapy improves health-related quality of life. *Respir Med*. 2004;98(4):285-293.

43.   Kamal AH, Maguire JM, Wheeler JL, Currow DC, Abernethy AP. Dyspnea review for the palliative care professional: treatment goals and therapeutic options. *J Palliat Med*. 2012;15(1):106-114.

44.   Abernethy AP, Currow DC, Frith P, Fazekas B. Prescribing palliative oxygen: a clinician survey of expected benefit and patterns of use. *Palliat Med*. 2005;19(2):168-170.

45.   Johnson MJ, Abernethy AP, Currow DC. The evidence base for oxygen for chronic refractory breathlessness: issues, gaps, and a future work plan. *J Pain Symptom Manage*. 2013;45(4):763-775.

46. Campbell ML, Yarandi H, Dove-Medows E. Oxygen is nonbeneficial for most patients who are near death. *J Pain Symptom Manage*. 2013;45(3):517-523.

47. Hardinge M, Annandale J, Bourne S, et al. British Thoracic Society guidelines for home oxygen use in adults. *Thorax*. 2015;70 Suppl 1:i1-43.

48. Lanken PN, Terry PB, Delisser HM, et al. An official American Thoracic Society clinical policy statement: palliative care for patients with respiratory diseases and critical illnesses. *Am J Respir Crit Care Med*. 2008;177(8):912-927.

49. Mahler DA, Selecky PA, Harrod CG, et al. American College of Chest Physicians consensus statement on the management of dyspnea in patients with advanced lung or heart disease. *Chest*. 2010;137(3):674-691.

50. Thomas JR, von Gunten CF. Management of dyspnea. *J Support Oncol*. 2003;1(1):23-32.

51. Del Fabbro E, Dalal S, Bruera E. Symptom control in palliative care—part III: dyspnea and delirium. *J Palliat Med*. 2006;9(2):422-436.

52. Campbell ML. Terminal dyspnea and respiratory distress. *Crit Care Clin*. 2004;20(3):403-417.

53. Light RW, Muro JR, Sato RI, Stansbury DW, Fischer CE, Brown SE. Effects of oral morphine on breathlessness and exercise tolerance in patients with chronic obstructive pulmonary disease. *Am Rev Respir Dis*. 1989;139(1):126-133.

54. Johnson MJ, McDonagh TA, Harkness A, McKay SE, Dargie HJ. Morphine for the relief of breathlessness in patients with chronic heart failure—a pilot study. *Eur J Heart Fail*. 2002;4(6):753-756.

55. Coyne PJ, Viswanathan R, Smith TJ. Nebulized fentanyl citrate improves patients' perception of breathing, respiratory rate, and oxygen saturation in dyspnea. *J Pain Symptom Manage*. 2002;23(2):157-160.

56. Barnes H, McDonald J, Smallwood N, Manser R. Opioids for the palliation of refractory breathlessness in adults with advanced disease and terminal illness. *Cochrane Database Syst Rev*. 2016;3:Cd011008.

57. Banzett RB, Adams L, O'Donnell CR, Gilman SA, Lansing RW, Schwartzstein RM. Using laboratory models to test treatment: morphine reduces dyspnea and hypercapnic ventilatory response. *Am J Respir Crit Care Med*. 2011.

58. Vargas-Bermudez A, Cardenal F, Porta-Sales J. Opioids for the management of dyspnea in cancer patients: evidence of the last 15 years—a systematic review. *J Pain Palliat Care Pharmacother*. 2015;29(4):341-352.

59. Bruera E, MacEachern T, Ripamonti C, Hanson J. Subcutaneous morphine for dyspnea in cancer patients. *Ann Intern Med*. 1993;119(9):906-907.

60. Abernethy AP, Currow DC, Frith P, Fazekas BS, McHugh A, Bui C. Randomised, double blind, placebo controlled crossover trial of sustained release morphine for the management of refractory dyspnoea. *BMJ*. 2003;327(7414):523-528.

61. Currow DC, McDonald C, Oaten S, et al. Once-daily opioids for chronic dyspnea: a dose increment and pharmacovigilance study. *J Pain Symptom Manage*. 2011;42(3):388-399.

62. Bausewein C, Simon ST. Inhaled nebulized and intranasal opioids for the relief of breathlessness. *Curr Opin Support Palliat Care*. 2014;8(3):208-212.

63. Charles MA, Reymond L, Israel F. Relief of incident dyspnea in palliative cancer patients: a pilot, randomized, controlled trial comparing nebulized hydromorphone, systemic hydromorphone, and nebulized saline. *J Pain Symptom Manage*. 2008;36(1):29-38.

64. Clemens KE, Quednau I, Klaschik E. Is there a higher risk of respiratory depression in opioid-naive palliative care patients during symptomatic therapy of dyspnea with strong opioids? *J Palliat Med*. 2008;11(2):204-216.

65. Clemens KE, Klaschik E. Symptomatic therapy of dyspnea with strong opioids and its effect on ventilation in palliative care patients. *J Pain Symptom Manage*. 2007;33(4):473-481.

66. Lopez-Saca JM, Centeno C. Opioids prescription for symptoms relief and the impact on respiratory function: updated evidence. *Curr Opin Support Palliat Care.* 2014;8(4):383-390.

67. Dunwoody CJ, Arnold R. Fast facts and concepts # 39: using Naloxone. *Fast Facts and Concepts.* 2015. https://www.mypcnow.org/blank-fnbfg. Accessed July 10, 2017.

68. Dahan A, Aarts L, Smith TW. Incidence, reversal, and prevention of opioid-induced respiratory depression. *Anesthesiology.* 2010;112(1):226-238.

69. Simon ST, Higginson IJ, Booth S, Harding R, Bausewein C. Benzodiazepines for the relief of breathlessness in advanced malignant and non-malignant diseases in adults. *Cochrane Database Syst Rev.* 2010(1):Cd007354.

70. Simon ST, Higginson IJ, Booth S, Harding R, Weingartner V, Bausewein C. Benzodiazepines for the relief of breathlessness in advanced malignant and non-malignant diseases in adults. *Cochrane Database Syst Rev.* 2016;10:Cd007354.

71. Navigante AH, Castro MA, Cerchietti LC. Morphine versus midazolam as upfront therapy to control dyspnea perception in cancer patients while its underlying cause is sought or treated. *J Pain Symptom Manage.* 2010;39(5):820-830.

72. Ekstrom MP, Bornefalk-Hermansson A, Abernethy AP, Currow DC. Safety of benzodiazepines and opioids in very severe respiratory disease: national prospective study. *BMJ.* 2014;348:g445.

73. US Food and Drug Administration. New safety measures announced for opioid analgesics, prescription opioid cough products, and benzodiazepines. 2016; https://www.fda.gov/Drugs/DrugSafety/InformationbyDrugClass/ucm518110.htm. Accessed July 10, 2017.

74. Clemens KE, Klaschik E. Dyspnoea associated with anxiety-symptomatic therapy with opioids in combination with lorazepam and its effect on ventilation in palliative care patients. *Support Care Cancer.* 2010;19(12):2027-2033.

75. Navigante AH, Cerchietti LC, Castro MA, Lutteral MA, Cabalar ME. Midazolam as adjunct therapy to morphine in the alleviation of severe dyspnea perception in patients with advanced cancer. *J Pain Symptom Manage.* 2006;31(1):38-47.

76. Zacharias H, Raw J, Nunn A, Parsons S, Johnson M. Is there a role for subcutaneous furosemide in the community and hospice management of end-stage heart failure? *Palliat Med.* 2011;25(6):658-663.

77. Campbell ML, Yarandi HN. Death rattle is not associated with patient respiratory distress: is pharmacologic treatment indicated? *J Palliat Med.* 2013;16(10):1255-1259.

78. Mercadante S, Villari P, Ferrera P. Refractory death rattle: deep aspiration facilitates the effects of antisecretory agents. *J Pain Symptom Manage.* 2011;41(3):637-639.

79. Wee B, Hillier R. Interventions for noisy breathing in patients near to death. *Cochrane Database Syst Rev.* 2008(1):CD005177.

80. Pan CX, Morrison RS, Ness J, Fugh-Berman A, Leipzig RM. Complementary and alternative medicine in the management of pain, dyspnea, and nausea and vomiting near the end of life. A systematic review. *J Pain Symptom Manage.* 2000;20(5):374-387.

81. Vickers AJ, Feinstein MB, Deng GE, Cassileth BR. Acupuncture for dyspnea in advanced cancer: a randomized, placebo-controlled pilot trial [ISRCTN89462491]. *BMC Palliat Care.* 2005;4:5.

82. Lewith GT, Prescott P, Davis CL. Can a standardized acupuncture technique palliate disabling breathlessness: a single-blind, placebo-controlled crossover study. *Chest.* 2004;125(5):1783-1790.

83. Suzuki M, Namura K, Ohno Y, et al. The effect of acupuncture in the treatment of chronic obstructive pulmonary disease. *J Altern Complement Med.* 2008;14(9):1097-1105.

84. Suzuki M, Muro S, Ando Y, et al. A randomized, placebo-controlled trial of acupuncture in patients with chronic obstructive pulmonary disease (COPD): the COPD-acupuncture trial (CAT). *Arch Intern Med.* 2012;172(11):878-886.

85. Roca O, Riera J, Torres F, Masclans JR. High-flow oxygen therapy in acute respiratory failure. *Respir Care*. 2010;55(4):408-413.

86. Hillberg RE, Johnson DC. Noninvasive ventilation. *N Engl J Med*. 1997;337(24):1746-1752.

87. Heinemann F, Budweiser S, Jorres RA, et al. The role of non-invasive home mechanical ventilation in patients with chronic obstructive pulmonary disease requiring prolonged weaning. *Respirology*. 2011;16(8):1273-1280.

88. Diaz GG, Alcaraz AC, Talavera JC, et al. Noninvasive positive-pressure ventilation to treat hypercapnic coma secondary to respiratory failure. *Chest*. 2005;127(3):952-960.

89. Kleopa KA, Sherman M, Neal B, Romano GJ, Heiman-Patterson T. BiPAP improves survival and rate of pulmonary function decline in patients with ALS. *J Neurol Sci*. 1999;164(1):82-88.

90. Eisen A. Amyotrophic lateral sclerosis: a 40-year personal perspective. *J Clin Neurosci*. 2009;16(4):505-512.

91. Yeow ME, Santanilla JI. Noninvasive positive pressure ventilation in the emergency department. *Emerg Med Clin North Am*. 2008;26(3):835-847.

92. Hui D, Morgado M, Chisholm G, et al. High-flow oxygen and bilevel positive airway pressure for persistent dyspnea in patients with advanced cancer: a phase II randomized trial. *J Pain Symptom Manage*. 2013;46(4):463-473.

93. Quill CM, Quill TE. Palliative use of noninvasive ventilation: navigating murky waters. *J Palliat Med*. 2014;17(6):657-661.

94. Curtis JR, Cook DJ, Sinuff T, et al. Noninvasive positive pressure ventilation in critical and palliative care settings: understanding the goals of therapy. *Crit Care Med*. 2007;35(3):932-939.

95. Smith I, Nadig V, Lasserson TJ. Educational, supportive and behavioural interventions to improve usage of continuous positive airway pressure machines for adults with obstructive sleep apnoea. *Cochrane Database Syst Rev*. 2009(2):CD007736.

96. Billings JA, Block SD. Part III: a guide for structured discussions. *J Palliat Med*. 2011;14(9):1058-1064.

97. Quill TE, Lo B, Brock DW, Meisel A. Last-resort options for palliative sedation. *Ann Intern Med*. 2009;151(6):421-424.

98. Billings JA. The end-of-life family meeting in intensive care part I: indications, outcomes, and family needs. *J Palliat Med*. 2011;14(9):1042-1050.

99. Shanawani H, Wenrich MD, Tonelli MR, Curtis JR. Meeting physicians' responsibilities in providing end-of-life care. *Chest*. 2008;133(3):775-786.

100. Schneiderman LJ, Gilmer T, Teetzel HD, et al. Effect of ethics consultations on nonbeneficial life-sustaining treatments in the intensive care setting: a randomized controlled trial. *JAMA*. 2003;290(9):1166-1172.

101. Truog RD, Cist AF, Brackett SE, et al. Recommendations for end-of-life care in the intensive care unit: The Ethics Committee of the Society of Critical Care Medicine. *Crit Care Med*. 2001;29(12):2332-2348.

102. Szalados JE. Discontinuation of mechanical ventilation at end-of-life: the ethical and legal boundaries of physician conduct in termination of life support. *Crit Care Clin*. 2007;23(2):317-337, xi.

103. Marr L, Weissman DE. Withdrawal of ventilatory support from the dying adult patient. *J Support Oncol*. 2004;2(3):283-288.

104. Treece PD, Engelberg RA, Crowley L, et al. Evaluation of a standardized order form for the withdrawal of life support in the intensive care unit. *Crit Care Med*. 2004;32(5):1141-1148.

105. Rubenfeld GD. Principles and practice of withdrawing life-sustaining treatments. *Crit Care Clin*. 2004;20(3):435-451, ix.

106. Ikeda M, Aiba T, Ikui A, et al. Taste disorders: a survey of the examination methods and treatments used in Japan. *Acta Otolaryngol*. 2005;125(11):1203-1210.

107. Halyard MY, Jatoi A, Sloan JA, et al. Does zinc sulfate prevent therapy-induced taste alterations in head and neck cancer patients? Results of phase III double-blind, placebo-controlled trial from the North Central Cancer Treatment Group (N01C4). *Int J Radiat Oncol Biol Phys.* 2007;67(5):1318-1322.

108. Skoretz SA, Flowers HL, Martino R. The incidence of dysphagia following endotracheal intubation: a systematic review. *Chest.* 2010;137(3):665-673.

109. Bogaardt H, Veerbeek L, Kelly K, van der Heide A, van Zuylen L, Speyer R. Swallowing problems at the end of the palliative phase: incidence and severity in 164 unsedated patients. *Dysphagia.* 2015;30(2):145-151.

110. Pace A, Di Lorenzo C, Guariglia L, Jandolo B, Carapella CM, Pompili A. End of life issues in brain tumor patients. *J Neurooncol.* 2009;91(1):39-43.

111. Meurman JH, Gronroos L. Oral and dental health care of oral cancer patients: hyposalivation, caries and infections. *Oral Oncol.* 2010;46(6):464-467.

112. Rieger JM, Jha N, Lam Tang JA, Harris J, Seikaly H. Functional outcomes related to the prevention of radiation-induced xerostomia: oral pilocarpine versus submandibular salivary gland transfer. *Head Neck.* 2011.

113. Deasy JO, Moiseenko V, Marks L, Chao KS, Nam J, Eisbruch A. Radiotherapy dose-volume effects on salivary gland function. *Int J Radiat Oncol Biol Phys.* 2010;76(3 Suppl):S58-63.

114. Burlage FR, Roesink JM, Kampinga HH, et al. Protection of salivary function by concomitant pilocarpine during radiotherapy: a double-blind, randomized, placebo-controlled study. *Int J Radiat Oncol Biol Phys.* 2008;70(1):14-22.

115. Miller LJ. Oral pilocarpine for radiation-induced xerostomia. *Cancer Bull.* 1993;45(6):549-550.

116. Davies AN. A comparison of artificial saliva and chewing gum in the management of xerostomia in patients with advanced cancer. *Palliat Med.* 2000;14(3):197-203.

117. Regnard C, Allport S, Stephenson L. ABC of palliative care. Mouth care, skin care, and lymphoedema. *BMJ.* 1997;315(7114):1002-1005.

118. Wolff A, Joshi RK, Ekstrom J, et al. A guide to medications inducing salivary gland dysfunction, xerostomia, and subjective sialorrhea: s systematic review sponsored by the World Workshop on Oral Medicine VI. *Drugs R D.* 2017;17(1):1-28.

119. Mercadante S, Calderone L, Villari P, et al. The use of pilocarpine in opioid-induced xerostomia. *Palliat Med.* 2000;14(6):529-531.

120. Pappas PG, Kauffman CA, Andes DR, et al. Clinical practice guideline for the management of candidiasis: 2016 update by the Infectious Diseases Society of America. *Clin Infect Dis.* 2016;62(4):e1-50.

121. Glenny AM, Fernandez Mauleffinch LM, Pavitt S, Walsh T. Interventions for the prevention and treatment of herpes simplex virus in patients being treated for cancer. *Cochrane Database Syst Rev.* 2009(1):CD006706.

122. Nozaki-Taguchi N, Shutoh M, Shimoyama N. Potential utility of peripherally applied loperamide in oral chronic graft-versus-host disease related pain. *Jpn J Clin Oncol.* 2008;38(12):857-860.

123. Epstein JB, Epstein JD, Epstein MS, Oien H, Truelove EL. Oral doxepin rinse: the analgesic effect and duration of pain reduction in patients with oral mucositis due to cancer therapy. *Anesth Analg.* 2006;103(2):465-470, table of contents.

124. Ryan AJ, Lin F, Atayee RS. Ketamine mouthwash for mucositis pain. *J Palliat Med.* 2009;12(11):989-991.

125. Gairard-Dory AC, Schaller C, Mennecier B, et al. Chemoradiotherapy-induced esophagitis pain relieved by topical morphine: three cases. *J Pain Symptom Manage.* 2005;30(2):107-109.

126. Ellershaw JE, Sutcliffe JM, Saunders CM. Dehydration and the dying patient. *J Pain Symptom Manage.* 1995;10(3):192-197.

127. Javle M, Ailawadhi S, Yang GY, Nwogu CE, Schiff MD, Nava HR. Palliation of malignant dysphagia in esophageal cancer: a literature-based review. *J Support Oncol.* 2006;4(8):365-373, 379.

128. Sundelof M, Ringby D, Stockeld D, Granstrom L, Jonas E, Freedman J. Palliative treatment of malignant dysphagia with self-expanding metal stents: a 12-year experience. *Scand J Gastroenterol.* 2007;42(1):11-16.

129. Papachristou GI, Baron TH. Use of stents in benign and malignant esophageal disease. *Rev Gastroenterol Disord.* 2007;7(2):74-88.

130. Bergquist H, Johnsson E, Nyman J, et al. Combined stent insertion and single high-dose brachytherapy in patients with advanced esophageal cancer—results of a prospective safety study. *Dis Esophagus.* 2011;25(5):410-415.

131. Diamantis G, Scarpa M, Bocus P, et al. Quality of life in patients with esophageal stenting for the palliation of malignant dysphagia. *World J Gastroenterol.* 2011;17(2):144-150.

132. Grilo A, Santos CA, Fonseca J. Percutaneous endoscopic gastrostomy for nutritional palliation of upper esophageal cancer unsuitable for esophageal stenting. *Arq Gastroenterol.* 2012;49(3):227-231.

133. Silani V, Kasarskis EJ, Yanagisawa N. Nutritional management in amyotrophic lateral sclerosis: a worldwide perspective. *J Neurol.* 1998;245 Suppl 2:S13-19; discussion S29.

134. Multi-Society Task Force on PVS. Medical aspects of the persistent vegetative state (2). *N Engl J Med.* 1994;330(22):1572-1579.

135. Danis M. Stopping artificial nutrition and hydration at the end of life. *UpToDate.* 2016. https://www.uptodate.com/contents/stopping-artificial-nutrition-and-hydration-at-the-end-of-life. Accessed July 5, 2017.

136. Borum ML, Lynn J, Zhong Z, et al. The effect of nutritional supplementation on survival in seriously ill hospitalized adults: an evaluation of the SUPPORT data. Study to Understand Prognoses and Preferences for Outcomes and Risks of Treatments. *J Am Geriatr Soc.* 2000;48(5 Suppl):S33-38.

137. Jatoi A, Loprinzi CL. The role of parenteral and enteral/oral nutritional support in patients with cancer. *UpToDate.* 2016. https://www.uptodate.com/contents/the-role-of-parenteral-and-enteral-oral-nutritional-support-in-patients-with-cancer. Accessed July 6, 2017.

138. Gillick MR. Rethinking the role of tube feeding in patients with advanced dementia. *N Engl J Med.* 2000;342(3):206-210.

139. American Geriatrics Society Ethics Committee and Clinical Practice and Models of Care Committee. American Geriatrics Society feeding tubes in advanced dementia position statement. *J Am Geriatr Soc.* 2014;62(8):1590-1593.

140. Gomes CA, Jr., Lustosa SA, Matos D, Andriolo RB, Waisberg DR, Waisberg J. Percutaneous endoscopic gastrostomy versus nasogastric tube feeding for adults with swallowing disturbances. *Cochrane Database Syst Rev.* 2010(11):CD008096.

141. Remington R, Hultman T. Hypodermoclysis to treat dehydration: a review of the evidence. *J Am Geriatr Soc.* 2007;55(12):2051-2055.

142. Akbar U, Dham B, He Y, et al. Incidence and mortality trends of aspiration pneumonia in Parkinson's disease in the United States, 1979-2010. *Parkinsonism Relat Disord.* 2015;21(9):1082-1086.

143. Fortunati N, Manti R, Birocco N, et al. Pro-inflammatory cytokines and oxidative stress/antioxidant parameters characterize the bio-humoral profile of early cachexia in lung cancer patients. *Oncol Rep.* 2007;18(6):1521-1527.

144. Johnen H, Lin S, Kuffner T, et al. Tumor-induced anorexia and weight loss are mediated by the TGF-beta superfamily cytokine MIC-1. *Nat Med.* 2007;13(11):1333-1340.

145. Buchanan JB, Johnson RW. Regulation of food intake by inflammatory cytokines in the brain. *Neuroendocrinology.* 2007;86(3):183-190.

146. Fearon K, Strasser F, Anker SD, et al. Definition and classification of cancer cachexia: an international consensus. *Lancet Oncol.* 2011;12(5):489-495.

147. Ali S, Garcia JM. Sarcopenia, cachexia and aging: diagnosis, mechanisms and therapeutic options—a mini-review. *Gerontology*. 2014;60(4):294-305.

148. Evans WJ. Skeletal muscle loss: cachexia, sarcopenia, and inactivity. *Am J Clin Nutr*. 2010;91(4):1123s-1127s.

149. Fearon KC. Cancer cachexia and fat-muscle physiology. *N Engl J Med*. 2011;365(6):565-567.

150. McMahon MM, Hurley DL, Kamath PS, Mueller PS. Medical and ethical aspects of long-term enteral tube feeding. *Mayo Clin Proc*. 2005;80(11):1461-1476.

151. Dahele M, Fearon KC. Research methodology: cancer cachexia syndrome. *Palliat Med*. 2004;18(5):409-417.

152. Arner P. Medicine. Lipases in cachexia. *Science*. 2011;333(6039):163-164.

153. Balkwill F, Mantovani A. Inflammation and cancer: back to Virchow? *Lancet*. 2001;357(9255):539-545.

154. Prado CM, Baracos VE, McCargar LJ, et al. Sarcopenia as a determinant of chemotherapy toxicity and time to tumor progression in metastatic breast cancer patients receiving capecitabine treatment. *Clin Cancer Res*. 2009;15(8):2920-2926.

155. LeBlanc TW, Nipp RD, Rushing CN, et al. Correlation between the international consensus definition of the Cancer Anorexia-Cachexia Syndrome (CACS) and patient-centered outcomes in advanced non-small cell lung cancer. *J Pain Symptom Manage*. 2015;49(4):680-689.

156. Del Fabbro E, Hui D, Dalal S, Dev R, Noorhuddin Z, Bruera E. Clinical outcomes and contributors to weight loss in a cancer cachexia clinic. *J Palliat Med*. 2011;14(9):1004-1008.

157. Bruera E, Belzile M, Neumann C, Harsanyi Z, Babul N, Darke A. A double-blind, crossover study of controlled-release metoclopramide and placebo for the chronic nausea and dyspepsia of advanced cancer. *J Pain Symptom Manage*. 2000;19(6):427-435.

158. Riechelmann RP, Burman D, Tannock IF, Rodin G, Zimmermann C. Phase II trial of mirtazapine for cancer-related cachexia and anorexia. *Am J Hosp Palliat Care*. 2010;27(2):106-110.

159. Popiela T, Lucchi R, Giongo F. Methylprednisolone as palliative therapy for female terminal cancer patients. The Methylprednisolone Female Preterminal Cancer Study Group. *Eur J Cancer Clin Oncol*. 1989;25(12):1823-1829.

160. Yamagishi A, Morita T, Miyashita M, Sato K, Tsuneto S, Shima Y. The care strategy for families of terminally ill cancer patients who become unable to take nourishment orally: recommendations from a nationwide survey of bereaved family members' experiences. *J Pain Symptom Manage*. 2010;40(5):671-683.

161. Ruiz Garcia V, Lopez-Briz E, Carbonell Sanchis R, Gonzalvez Perales JL, Bort-Marti S. Megestrol acetate for treatment of anorexia-cachexia syndrome. *Cochrane Database Syst Rev*. 2013(3):Cd004310.

162. Berenstein EG, Ortiz Z. Megestrol acetate for the treatment of anorexia-cachexia syndrome. *Cochrane Database Syst Rev*. 2005(2):CD004310.

163. Tisdale MJ. Clinical anticachexia treatments. *Nutr Clin Pract*. 2006;21(2):168-174.

164. Bruera E, Macmillan K, Kuehn N, Hanson J, MacDonald RN. A controlled trial of megestrol acetate on appetite, caloric intake, nutritional status, and other symptoms in patients with advanced cancer. *Cancer*. 1990;66(6):1279-1282.

165. Von Roenn JH, Armstrong D, Kotler DP, et al. Megestrol acetate in patients with AIDS-related cachexia. *Ann Intern Med*. 1994;121(6):393-399.

166. Campbell TC, Von Roenn JH. Anorexia/weight loss. In: Berger AM, Shuster JL, Von Roenn JH, eds. *Principles and Practice of Palliative Care and Supportive Oncology*. 3rd ed. Philadelphia, PA: Lippincott Williams & Wilkins; 2007:125-130.

167. Reuben DB, Hirsch SH, Zhou K, Greendale GA. The effects of megestrol acetate suspension for elderly patients with reduced appetite after hospitalization: a phase II randomized clinical trial. *J Am Geriatr Soc*. 2005;53(6):970-975.

168. American Geriatrics Society Beers Criteria Update Expert Panel. American Geriatrics Society 2015 updated Beers Criteria for Potentially Inappropriate Medication Use in Older Adults. *J Am Geriatr Soc.* 2015;63(11):2227-2246.

169. Naing A, Dalal S, Abdelrahim M, et al. Olanzapine for cachexia in patients with advanced cancer: an exploratory study of effects on weight and metabolic cytokines. *Support Care Cancer.* 2015;23(9):2649-2654.

170. Navari RM, Brenner MC. Treatment of cancer-related anorexia with olanzapine and megestrol acetate: a randomized trial. *Support Care Cancer.* 2010;18(8):951-956.

171. Miller S, McNutt L, McCann MA, McCorry N. Use of corticosteroids for anorexia in palliative medicine: a systematic review. *J Palliat Med.* 2014;17(4):482-485.

172. Moses AW, Slater C, Preston T, Barber MD, Fearon KC. Reduced total energy expenditure and physical activity in cachectic patients with pancreatic cancer can be modulated by an energy and protein dense oral supplement enriched with n-3 fatty acids. *Br J Cancer.* 2004;90(5):996-1002.

173. Ries A, Trottenberg P, Elsner F, et al. A systematic review on the role of fish oil for the treatment of cachexia in advanced cancer: an EPCRC cachexia guidelines project. *Palliat Med.* 2011;26(4):294-304.

174. Davis M, Lasheen W, Walsh D, Mahmoud F, Bicanovsky L, Lagman R. A phase II dose titration study of thalidomide for cancer-associated anorexia. *J Pain Symptom Manage.* 2011;43(1):78-86.

175. Beal JE, Olson R, Laubenstein L, et al. Dronabinol as a treatment for anorexia associated with weight loss in patients with AIDS. *J Pain Symptom Manage.* 1995;10(2):89-97.

176. Aggarwal SK, Carter GT, Sullivan MD, ZumBrunnen C, Morrill R, Mayer JD. Medicinal use of cannabis in the United States: historical perspectives, current trends, and future directions. *J Opioid Manag.* 2009;5(3):153-168.

177. Whiting PF, Wolff RF, Deshpande S, et al. Cannabinoids for medical use: a systematic review and meta-analysis. *JAMA.* 2015;313(24):2456-2473.

178. Strasser F, Luftner D, Possinger K, et al. Comparison of orally administered cannabis extract and delta-9-tetrahydrocannabinol in treating patients with cancer-related anorexia-cachexia syndrome: a multicenter, phase III, randomized, double-blind, placebo-controlled clinical trial from the Cannabis-In-Cachexia Study Group. *J Clin Oncol.* 2006;24(21):3394-3400.

179. Temel JS, Abernethy AP, Currow DC, et al. Anamorelin in patients with non-small-cell lung cancer and cachexia (ROMANA 1 and ROMANA 2): results from two randomised, double-blind, phase 3 trials. *Lancet Oncol.* 2016;17(4):519-531.

180. Berger AM, Mooney K, Banerjee C, et al. NCCN Clinical Practice Guidelines in Oncology (NCCN Guidelines): Cancer-Related Fatigue. Fort Washington, PA: National Comprehensive Cancer Network; 2017. https://www.nccn.org/professionals/physician_gls/pdf/fatigue.pdf. Accessed July 6, 2017.

181. Markowitz AJ, Rabow MW. Palliative management of fatigue at the close of life: "it feels like my body is just worn out". *JAMA.* 2007;298(2):217.

182. Mucke M, Cuhls H, Peuckmann-Post V, Minton O, Stone P, Radbruch L. Pharmacological treatments for fatigue associated with palliative care. *Cochrane Database Syst Rev.* 2015;(5):Cd006788.

183. Piper BF, Cella D. Cancer-related fatigue: definitions and clinical subtypes. *J Natl Compr Canc Netw.* 2010;8(8):958-966.

184. Vogl D, Rosenfeld B, Breitbart W, et al. Symptom prevalence, characteristics, and distress in AIDS outpatients. *J Pain Symptom Manage.* 1999;18(4):253-262.

185. Kutner JS, Kassner CT, Nowels DE. Symptom burden at the end of life: hospice providers' perceptions. *J Pain Symptom Manage.* 2001;21(6):473-480.

186. Poort H, Peters ME, Gielissen MF, et al. Fatigue in advanced cancer patients: congruence between patients and their informal caregivers about patients' fatigue severity during cancer treatment with palliative intent and predictors of agreement. *J Pain Symptom Manage*. 2016;52(3):336-344.

187. Radbruch L, Strasser F, Elsner F, et al. Fatigue in palliative care patients—an EAPC approach. *Palliat Med*. 2008;22(1):13-32.

188. Whitehead LC, Unahi K, Burrell B, Crowe MT. The experience of fatigue across long-term conditions: A qualitative meta-synthesis. *J Pain Symptom Manage*. 2016;52(1):131-143, e131.

189. Blundell S, Ray KK, Buckland M, White PD. Chronic fatigue syndrome and circulating cytokines: a systematic review. *Brain Behav Immun*. 2015;50:186-195.

190. Watanabe SM, Nekolaichuk CL, Beaumont C. The Edmonton Symptom Assessment System, a proposed tool for distress screening in cancer patients: development and refinement. *Psychooncology*. 2012;21(9):977-985.

191. Lane TJ, Matthews DA, Manu P. The low yield of physical examinations and laboratory investigations of patients with chronic fatigue. *Am J Med Sci*. 1990;299(5):313-318.

192. Rao AV, Cohen HJ. Fatigue in older cancer patients: etiology, assessment, and treatment. *Semin Oncol*. 2008;35(6):633-642.

193. Dev R, Hui D, Dalal S, et al. Association between serum cortisol and testosterone levels, opioid therapy, and symptom distress in patients with advanced cancer. *J Pain Symptom Manage*. 2011;41(4):788-795.

194. Del Fabbro E, Hui D, Dalal S, Dev R, Nooruddin ZI, Bruera E. Clinical outcomes and contributors to weight loss in a cancer cachexia clinic. *J Palliat Med*. 2011;14(9):1004-1008.

195. Strasser F, Palmer JL, Schover LR, et al. The impact of hypogonadism and autonomic dysfunction on fatigue, emotional function, and sexual desire in male patients with advanced cancer: a pilot study. *Cancer*. 2006;107(12):2949-2957.

196. Fritschi C, Quinn L. Fatigue in patients with diabetes: a review. *J Psychosom Res*. 2010;69(1):33-41.

197. Munch TN, Zhang T, Willey J, Palmer JL, Bruera E. The association between anemia and fatigue in patients with advanced cancer receiving palliative care. *J Palliat Med*. 2005;8(6):1144-1149.

198. Bansal AS, Bradley AS, Bishop KN, Kiani-Alikhan S, Ford B. Chronic fatigue syndrome, the immune system and viral infection. *Brain Behav Immun*. 2012;26(1):24-31.

199. Miller KK, Perlis RH, Papakostas GI, et al. Low-dose transdermal testosterone augmentation therapy improves depression severity in women. *CNS Spectr*. 2009;14(12):688-694.

200. Matthews EE, Tanner JM, Dumont NA. Sleep disturbances in acutely ill patients with cancer. *Crit Care Nurs Clin North Am*. 2016;28(2):253-268.

201. Oldervoll LM, Loge JH, Paltiel H, et al. The effect of a physical exercise program in palliative care: a phase II study. *J Pain Symptom Manage*. 2006;31(5):421-430.

202. Mayo NE, Moriello C, Scott SC, Dawes D, Auais M, Chasen M. Pedometer-facilitated walking intervention shows promising effectiveness for reducing cancer fatigue: a pilot randomized trial. *Clin Rehabil*. 2014;28(12):1198-1209.

203. Cramp F, Byron-Daniel J. Exercise for the management of cancer-related fatigue in adults. *Cochrane Database Syst Rev*. 2012;11:Cd006145.

204. Puetz TW, Herring MP. Differential effects of exercise on cancer-related fatigue during and following treatment: a meta-analysis. *Am J Prev Med*. 2012;43(2):e1-24.

205. Brown JC, Huedo-Medina TB, Pescatello LS, Pescatello SM, Ferrer RA, Johnson BT. Efficacy of exercise interventions in modulating cancer-related fatigue among adult cancer survivors: a meta-analysis. *Cancer Epidemiol Biomarkers Prev*. 2011;20(1):123-133.

206. Strasser B, Steindorf K, Wiskemann J, Ulrich CM. Impact of resistance training in cancer survivors: a meta-analysis. *Med Sci Sports Exerc.* 2013;45(11):2080-2090.

207. Pinto BM, Frierson GM, Rabin C, Trunzo JJ, Marcus BH. Home-based physical activity intervention for breast cancer patients. *J Clin Oncol.* 2005;23(15):3577-3587.

208. Galvao DA, Newton RU. Review of exercise intervention studies in cancer patients. *J Clin Oncol.* 2005;23(4):899-909.

209. Lowe SS, Tan M, Faily J, Watanabe SM, Courneya KS. Physical activity in advanced cancer patients: a systematic review protocol. *Syst Rev.* 2016;5:43.

210. Gielissen MF, Verhagen CA, Bleijenberg G. Cognitive behaviour therapy for fatigued cancer survivors: long-term follow-up. *Br J Cancer.* 2007;97(5):612-618.

211. Gielissen MF, Verhagen S, Witjes F, Bleijenberg G. Effects of cognitive behavior therapy in severely fatigued disease-free cancer patients compared with patients waiting for cognitive behavior therapy: a randomized controlled trial. *J Clin Oncol.* 2006;24(30):4882-4887.

212. Yun YH, Lee KS, Kim YW, et al. Web-based tailored education program for disease-free cancer survivors with cancer-related fatigue: a randomized controlled trial. *J Clin Oncol.* 2012;30(12):1296-1303.

213. Bower JE. Cancer-related fatigue—mechanisms, risk factors, and treatments. *Nat Rev Clin Oncol.* 2014;11(10):597-609.

214. Bruera E, Valero V, Driver L, et al. Patient-controlled methylphenidate for cancer fatigue: a double-blind, randomized, placebo-controlled trial. *J Clin Oncol.* 2006;24(13):2073-2078.

215. Butler JM, Jr., Case LD, Atkins J, et al. A phase III, double-blind, placebo-controlled prospective randomized clinical trial of d-threo-methylphenidate HCl in brain tumor patients receiving radiation therapy. *Int J Radiat Oncol Biol Phys.* 2007;69(5):1496-1501.

216. Rammohan KW, Rosenberg JH, Lynn DJ, Blumenfeld AM, Pollak CP, Nagaraja HN. Efficacy and safety of modafinil (Provigil) for the treatment of fatigue in multiple sclerosis: a two centre phase 2 study. *J Neurol Neurosurg Psychiatry.* 2002;72(2):179-183.

217. Stankoff B, Waubant E, Confavreux C, et al. Modafinil for fatigue in MS: a randomized placebo-controlled double-blind study. *Neurology.* 2005;64(7):1139-1143.

218. Lange R, Volkmer M, Heesen C, Liepert J. Modafinil effects in multiple sclerosis patients with fatigue. *J Neurol.* 2009;256(4):645-650.

219. Murray TJ. Amantadine therapy for fatigue in multiple sclerosis. *Can J Neurol Sci.* 1985;12(3):251-254.

220. Krupp LB, Coyle PK, Doscher C, et al. Fatigue therapy in multiple sclerosis: results of a double-blind, randomized, parallel trial of amantadine, pemoline, and placebo. *Neurology.* 1995;45(11):1956-1961.

221. Ryan JL, Carroll JK, Ryan EP, Mustian KM, Fiscella K, Morrow GR. Mechanisms of cancer-related fatigue. *Oncologist.* 2007;12 Suppl 1:22-34.

222. Thornton LM, Andersen BL, Blakely WP. The pain, depression, and fatigue symptom cluster in advanced breast cancer: covariation with the hypothalamic-pituitary-adrenal axis and the sympathetic nervous system. *Health Psychol.* 2010;29(3):333-337.

223. Miaskowski C, Portenoy RK. Assessment and management of cancer-related fatigue. In: Berger AM, Shuster JL, von Roenn JH, eds. *Principles and Practices of Supportive Oncology.* 3rd ed. Philadelphia, PA: Lippincott, Williams & Wilkins; 2007:95-104.

224. Fisch MJ, Loehrer PJ, Kristeller J, et al. Fluoxetine versus placebo in advanced cancer outpatients: a double-blinded trial of the Hoosier Oncology Group. *J Clin Oncol.* 2003;21(10):1937-1943.

225. Reuben DB, Mor V. Nausea and vomiting in terminal cancer patients. *Arch Intern Med.* 1986;146(10):2021-2023.

226. Herrinton LJ, Neslund-Dudas C, Rolnick SJ, et al. Complications at the end of life in ovarian cancer. *J Pain Symptom Manage.* 2007;34(3):237-243.

227. Henry DH, Viswanathan HN, Elkin EP, Traina S, Wade S, Cella D. Symptoms and treatment burden associated with cancer treatment: results from a cross-sectional national survey in the US. *Support Care Cancer.* 2008;16(7):791-801.

228. Lichter I. Results of antiemetic management in terminal illness. *J Palliat Care.* 1993;9(2):19-21.

229. Garrett K, Tsuruta K, Walker S, Jackson S, Sweat M. Managing nausea and vomiting. Current strategies. *Crit Care Nurse.* 2003;23(1):31-50.

230. Stephenson J, Davies A. An assessment of aetiology-based guidelines for the management of nausea and vomiting in patients with advanced cancer. *Support Care Cancer.* 2006;14(4):348-353.

231. Bentley A, Boyd K. Use of clinical pictures in the management of nausea and vomiting: a prospective audit. *Palliat Med.* 2001;15(3):247-253.

232. Glare PA, Dunwoodie D, Clark K, et al. Treatment of nausea and vomiting in terminally ill cancer patients. *Drugs.* 2008;68(18):2575-2590.

233. Collis E, Mather H. Nausea and vomiting in palliative care. *BMJ.* 2015;351:h6249.

234. Ettinger DS, Berger MJ, Aston J, et al. NCCN Clincial Practice Guidleines in Oncology: Antiemesis. Fort Washington, PA: National Comprehensive Cancer Network; 2017. https://www.nccn.org/professionals/physician_gls/pdf/antiemesis.pdf. Accessed July 6, 2017.

235. Gralla RJ, Osoba D, Kris MG, et al. Recommendations for the use of antiemetics: evidence-based, clinical practice guidelines. American Society of Clinical Oncology. *J Clin Oncol.* 1999;17(9):2971-2994.

236. Billio A, Morello E, Clarke MJ. Serotonin receptor antagonists for highly emetogenic chemotherapy in adults. *Cochrane Database Syst Rev.* 2010(1):CD006272.

237. Hesketh PJ, Sanz-Altamira P, Bushey J, Hesketh AM. Prospective evaluation of the incidence of delayed nausea and vomiting in patients with colorectal cancer receiving oxaliplatin-based chemotherapy. *Support Care Cancer.* 2011;20(5):1043-1047.

238. Hesketh PJ, Van Belle S, Aapro M, et al. Differential involvement of neurotransmitters through the time course of cisplatin-induced emesis as revealed by therapy with specific receptor antagonists. *Eur J Cancer.* 2003;39(8):1074-1080.

239. Warr DG, Hesketh PJ, Gralla RJ, et al. Efficacy and tolerability of aprepitant for the prevention of chemotherapy-induced nausea and vomiting in patients with breast cancer after moderately emetogenic chemotherapy. *J Clin Oncol.* 2005;23(12):2822-2830.

240. Akechi T, Okuyama T, Endo C, et al. Anticipatory nausea among ambulatory cancer patients undergoing chemotherapy: prevalence, associated factors, and impact on quality of life. *Cancer Sci.* 2010;101(12):2596-2600.

241. Gordon P, LeGrand SB, Walsh D. Nausea and vomiting in advanced cancer. *Eur J Pharmacol.* 2014;722:187-191.

242. Ripamonti C, De Conno F, Ventafridda V, Rossi B, Baines MJ. Management of bowel obstruction in advanced and terminal cancer patients. *Ann Oncol.* 1993;4(1):15-21.

243. Jatoi A, Podratz KC, Gill P, Hartmann LC. Pathophysiology and palliation of inoperable bowel obstruction in patients with ovarian cancer. *J Support Oncol.* 2004;2(4):323-334; discussion 334-327.

244. Nellgard P, Bojo L, Cassuto J. Importance of vasoactive intestinal peptide and somatostatin for fluid losses in small-bowel obstruction. *Scand J Gastroenterol.* 1995;30(5):464-469.

245. Nellgard P, Cassuto J. Inflammation as a major cause of fluid losses in small-bowel obstruction. *Scand J Gastroenterol.* 1993;28(12):1035-1041.

246. Lund B, Hansen M, Lundvall F, Nielsen NC, Sorensen BL, Hansen HH. Intestinal obstruction in patients with advanced carcinoma of the ovaries treated with combination chemotherapy. *Surg Gynecol Obstet.* 1989;169(3):213-218.

247. McKee KY, Widera E. Habitual prescribing of laxatives—it's time to flush outdated protocols down the drain. *JAMA Internal Medicine.* 2016;176(8):1217-1219.

248. Rao SS, Go JT. Update on the management of constipation in the elderly: new treatment options. *Clin Interv Aging.* 2010;5:163-171.

249. Portenoy RK, Thomas J, Moehl Boatwright ML, et al. Subcutaneous methylnaltrexone for the treatment of opioid-induced constipation in patients with advanced illness: a double-blind, randomized, parallel group, dose-ranging study. *J Pain Symptom Manage.* 2008;35(5):458-468.

250. Davis MP, Furste A. Glycopyrrolate: a useful drug in the palliation of mechanical bowel obstruction. *J Pain Symptom Manage.* 1999;18(3):153-154.

251. Ripamonti CI, Easson AM, Gerdes H. Management of malignant bowel obstruction. *Eur J Cancer.* 2008;44(8):1105-1115.

252. Hisanaga T, Shinjo T, Morita T, et al. Multicenter prospective study on efficacy and safety of octreotide for inoperable malignant bowel obstruction. *Jpn J Clin Oncol.* 2010;40(8):739-745.

253. Currow DC, Quinn S, Agar M, et al. Double-blind, placebo-controlled, randomized trial of octreotide in malignant bowel obstruction. *J Pain Symptom Manage.* 2015;49(5):814-821.

254. Mangili G, Franchi M, Mariani A, et al. Octreotide in the management of bowel obstruction in terminal ovarian cancer. *Gynecol Oncol.* 1996;61(3):345-348.

255. Mercadante S, Spoldi E, Caraceni A, Maddaloni S, Simonetti MT. Octreotide in relieving gastrointestinal symptoms due to bowel obstruction. *Palliat Med.* 1993;7(4):295-299.

256. Raijmakers NJ, van Zuylen L, Costantini M, et al. Artificial nutrition and hydration in the last week of life in cancer patients. A systematic literature review of practices and effects. *Ann Oncol.* 2011;22(7):1478-1486.

257. Dauphine CE, Tan P, Beart RW, Jr., Vukasin P, Cohen H, Corman ML. Placement of self-expanding metal stents for acute malignant large-bowel obstruction: a collective review. *Ann Surg Oncol.* 2002;9(6):574-579.

258. Henry JC, Pouly S, Sullivan R, et al. A scoring system for the prognosis and treatment of malignant bowel obstruction. *Surgery.* 2012;152(4):747-756; discussion 756-747.

259. Paul Olson TJ, Pinkerton C, Brasel KJ, Schwarze ML. Palliative surgery for malignant bowel obstruction from carcinomatosis: a systematic review. *JAMA Surg.* 2014;149(4):383-392.

260. Meisner S, Gonzalez-Huix F, Vandervoort JG, et al. Self-expandable metal stents for relieving malignant colorectal obstruction: short-term safety and efficacy within 30 days of stent procedure in 447 patients. *Gastrointest Endosc.* 2011;74(4):876-884.

261. Lee HJ, Hong SP, Cheon JH, et al. Long-term outcome of palliative therapy for malignant colorectal obstruction in patients with unresectable metastatic colorectal cancers: endoscopic stenting versus surgery. *Gastrointest Endosc.* 2011;73(3):535-542.

262. Mackay CD, Craig W, Hussey JK, Loudon MA. Self-expanding metallic stents for large bowel obstruction. *Br J Surg.* 2011;98(11):1625-1629.

263. Fernandez-Esparrach G, Bordas JM, Giraldez MD, et al. Severe complications limit long-term clinical success of self-expanding metal stents in patients with obstructive colorectal cancer. *Am J Gastroenterol.* 2010;105(5):1087-1093.

264. Casarett DJ, Inouye SK. Diagnosis and management of delirium near the end of life. *Ann Intern Med.* 2001;135(1):32-40.

265. Young J, Inouye SK. Delirium in older people. *BMJ.* 2007;334(7598):842-846.

266. Tomasi CD, Grandi C, Salluh J, et al. Comparison of CAM-ICU and ICDSC for the detection of delirium in critically ill patients focusing on relevant clinical outcomes. *J Crit Care*. 2011;27(2):212-217.

267. Wada T, Wada M, Onishi H. Characteristics, interventions, and outcomes of misdiagnosed delirium in cancer patients. *Palliat Support Care*. 2010;8(2):125-131.

268. Inouye SK, Bogardus ST, Jr., Charpentier PA, et al. A multicomponent intervention to prevent delirium in hospitalized older patients. *N Engl J Med*. 1999;340(9):669-676.

269. Inouye SK, Charpentier PA. Precipitating factors for delirium in hospitalized elderly persons. Predictive model and interrelationship with baseline vulnerability. *JAMA*. 1996;275(11):852-857.

270. Hshieh TT, Yue J, Oh E, et al. Effectiveness of multicomponent nonpharmacological delirium interventions: a meta-analysis. *JAMA Intern Med*. 2015;175(4):512-520.

271. O'Mahony R, Murthy L, Akunne A, Young J. Synopsis of the National Institute for Health and Clinical Excellence guideline for prevention of delirium. *Ann Intern Med*. 2011;154(11):746-751.

272. National Institute for Health and Care Excellence. Delirium: diagnosis, prevention, and management. 2010; https://www.nice.org.uk/guidance/cg103. Accessed July 10, 2017.

273. Barraclough J. ABC of palliative care. Depression, anxiety, and confusion. *BMJ*. 1997;315(7119):1365-1368.

274. Devlin JW, Bhat S, Roberts RJ, Skrobik Y. Current perceptions and practices surrounding the recognition and treatment of delirium in the intensive care unit: a survey of 250 critical care pharmacists from eight states. *Ann Pharmacother*. 2011;45(10):1217-1229.

275. McAvay GJ, Van Ness PH, Bogardus ST, Jr., et al. Older adults discharged from the hospital with delirium: 1-year outcomes. *J Am Geriatr Soc*. 2006;54(8):1245-1250.

276. McCusker J, Cole M, Abrahamowicz M, Primeau F, Belzile E. Delirium predicts 12-month mortality. *Arch Intern Med*. 2002;162(4):457-463.

277. Roche V. Southwestern Internal Medicine Conference. Etiology and management of delirium. *Am J Med Sci*. 2003;325(1):20-30.

278. Grover S, Kumar V, Chakrabarti S. Comparative efficacy study of haloperidol, olanzapine and risperidone in delirium. *J Psychosom Res*. 2011;71(4):277-281.

279. Young J, Murthy L, Westby M, Akunne A, O'Mahony R. Diagnosis, prevention, and management of delirium: summary of NICE guidance. *BMJ*. 2010;341:c3704.

280. Lonergan E, Britton AM, Luxenberg J, Wyller T. Antipsychotics for delirium. *Cochrane Database Syst Rev*. 2007(2):CD005594.

281. Lonergan E, Luxenberg J, Areosa Sastre A. Benzodiazepines for delirium. *Cochrane Database Syst Rev*. 2009(4):CD006379.

282. Agar MR, Lawlor PG, Quinn S, et al. Efficacy of oral risperidone, haloperidol, or placebo for symptoms of delirium among patients in palliative care: a randomized clinical trial. *JAMA Intern Med*. 2017;177(1):34-42.

283. Sultzer DL, Davis SM, Tariot PN, et al. Clinical symptom responses to atypical antipsychotic medications in Alzheimer's disease: phase 1 outcomes from the CATIE-AD effectiveness trial. *Am J Psychiatry*. 2008;165(7):844-854.

284. Wang PS, Schneeweiss S, Avorn J, et al. Risk of death in elderly users of conventional vs. atypical antipsychotic medications. *N Engl J Med*. 2005;353(22):2335-2341.

285. Huybrechts KF, Brookhart MA, Rothman KJ, et al. Comparison of different approaches to confounding adjustment in a study on the association of antipsychotic medication with mortality in older nursing home patients. *Am J Epidemiol*. 2011;174(9):1089-1099.

286. Rabins PV, Lyketsos CG. Antipsychotic drugs in dementia: what should be made of the risks? *JAMA*. 2005;294(15):1963-1965.

287. Caraceni A, Zecca E, Martini C, et al. Palliative sedation at the end of life at a tertiary cancer center. *Support Care Cancer.* 2012;20(6):1299-1307.

288. Morita T, Tei Y, Inoue S. Agitated terminal delirium and association with partial opioid substitution and hydration. *J Palliat Med.* 2003;6(4):557-563.

289. Galanakis C, Mayo NE, Gagnon B. Assessing the role of hydration in delirium at the end of life. *Curr Opin Support Palliat Care.* 2011;5(2):169-173.

290. Lewis MA, Hendrickson AW, Moynihan TJ. Oncologic emergencies: pathophysiology, presentation, diagnosis, and treatment. *CA Cancer J Clin.* 2011;61(5):287-314.

291. Kennedy KS, Wilson JF. Malignant thyroid lymphoma presenting as acute airway obstruction. *Ear Nose Throat J.* 1992;71(8):350, 353-355.

292. Song JU, Park HY, Kim H, et al. Prognostic factors for bronchoscopic intervention in advanced lung or esophageal cancer patients with malignant airway obstruction. *Ann Thorac Med.* 2013;8(2):86-92.

293. Yamaguchi S, Fujii T, Yajima R, et al. Preoperative multidisciplinary management of airway obstruction by huge goiter with papillary thyroid cancer. *Am Surg.* 2011;77(5):E91-93.

294. Gompelmann D, Eberhardt R, Herth FJ. Advanced malignant lung disease: what the specialist can offer. *Respiration.* 2011;82(2):111-123.

295. Kennedy MP, Morice RC, Jimenez CA, Eapen GA. Treatment of bronchial airway obstruction using a rotating tip microdebrider: a case report. *J Cardiothorac Surg.* 2007;2:16.

296. Sudheendra D, Barth MM, Hegde U, Wilson WH, Wood BJ. Radiofrequency ablation of lymphoma. *Blood.* 2006;107(4):1624-1626.

297. Allison R, Moghissi K, Downie G, Dixon K. Photodynamic therapy (PDT) for lung cancer. *Photodiagnosis Photodyn Ther.* 2011;8(3):231-239.

298. Manali ED, Stathopoulos GT, Gildea TR, et al. High dose-rate endobronchial radiotherapy for proximal airway obstruction due to lung cancer: 8-year experience of a referral center. *Cancer Biother Radiopharm.* 2010;25(2):207-213.

299. Muto P, Ravo V, Panelli G, Liguori G, Fraioli G. High-dose rate brachytherapy of bronchial cancer: treatment optimization using three schemes of therapy. *Oncologist.* 2000;5(3):209-214.

300. Saji H, Furukawa K, Tsutsui H, et al. Outcomes of airway stenting for advanced lung cancer with central airway obstruction. *Interact Cardiovasc Thorac Surg.* 2010;11(4):425-428.

301. Refaat MM, Katz WE. Neoplastic pericardial effusion. *Clin Cardiol.* 2011;34(10):593-598.

302. Spodick D. Acute cardiac tamponade. *New Engl J Med.* 2003;349(7):684-690.

303. Roy CL, Minor MA, Brookhart MA, Choudhry NK. Does this patient with a pericardial effusion have cardiac tamponade? *JAMA.* 2007;297(16):1810-1818.

304. Hosokawa K, Nakajima Y. An evaluation of acute cardiac tamponade by transesophageal echocardiography. *Anesth Analg.* 2008;106(1):61-62.

305. Gumrukcuoglu HA, Odabasi D, Akdag S, Ekim H. Management of cardiac tamponade: a comperative study between echo-guided pericardiocentesis and surgery. A report of 100 patients. *Cardiol Res Pract.* 2011;2011:197838.

306. Sagrista-Sauleda J, Merce AS, Soler-Soler J. Diagnosis and management of pericardial effusion. *World J Cardiol.* 2011;3(5):135-143.

307. Little WC, Freeman GL. Pericardial disease. *Circulation.* 2006;113(12):1622-1632.

308. Wang HJ, Hsu KL, Chiang FT, Tseng CD, Tseng YZ, Liau CS. Technical and prognostic outcomes of double-balloon pericardiotomy for large malignancy-related pericardial effusions. *Chest.* 2002;122(3):893-899.

309. Rimmer J, Giddings CE, Vaz F, Brooks J, Hopper C. Management of vascular complications of head and neck cancer. *J Laryngol Otol.* 2012;126(2):111-115.

310. Prommer E. Management of bleeding in the terminally ill patient. *Hematology.* 2005;10(3):167-175.

311. Pereira J, Phan T. Management of bleeding in patients with advanced cancer. *Oncologist.* 2004;9(5):561-570.

312. Powitzky R, Vasan N, Krempl G, Medina J. Carotid blowout in patients with head and neck cancer. *Ann Otol Rhinol Laryngol.* 2010;119(7):476-484.

313. Lagman R, Walsh D, Day K. Oxidized cellulose dressings for persistent bleeding from a superficial malignant tumor. *Am J Hosp Palliat Care.* 2002;19(6):417-418.

314. Kalmadi S, Tiu R, Lowe C, Jin T, Kalaycio M. Epsilon aminocaproic acid reduces transfusion requirements in patients with thrombocytopenic hemorrhage. *Cancer.* 2006;107(1):136-140.

315. Anwar D, Schaad N, Mazzocato C. Aerosolized vasopressin is a safe and effective treatment for mild to moderate recurrent hemoptysis in palliative care patients. *J Pain Symptom Manage.* 2005;29(5):427-429.

316. Hedges A, Coons JC, Saul M, Smith RE. Clinical effectiveness and safety outcomes associated with prothrombin complex concentrates. *J Thromb Thrombolysis.* 2016;42(1):6-10.

317. Clines GA. Mechanisms and treatment of hypercalcemia of malignancy. *Curr Opin Endocrinol Diabetes Obes.* 2011.

318. Basso U, Maruzzo M, Roma A, Camozzi V, Luisetto G, Lumachi F. Malignant hypercalcemia. *Curr Med Chem.* 2011;18(23):3462-3467.

319. Stewart A. Hypercalcemia associated with cancer. *N Engl J Med.* 2005;352(352):373-379.

320. Samphao S, Eremin JM, Eremin O. Oncological emergencies: clinical importance and principles of management. *Eur J Cancer Care (Engl).* 2010;19(6):707-713.

321. Siddiqui F, Weissman DE. Fast facts and concepts #151: hypercalcemia of malignancy. *Fast Facts and Concepts.* 2010. https://www.mypcnow.org/blank-rmac2. Accessed July 10, 2017.

322. McCurdy MT, Shanholtz CB. Oncologic emergencies. *Crit Care Med.* 2012;40(7):2212-2222.

323. Pi J, Kang Y, Smith M, Earl M, Norigian Z, McBride A. A review in the treatment of oncologic emergencies. *J Oncol Pharm Pract.* 2016;22(4):625-638.

324. Otto S, Schreyer C, Hafner S, et al. Bisphosphonate-related osteonecrosis of the jaws. Characteristics, risk factors, clinical features, localization and impact on oncological treatment. *J Craniomaxillofac Surg.* 2012;40(4):303-309.

325. Ruggiero SL, Dodson TB, Assael LA, Landesberg R, Marx RE, Mehrotra B. American Association of Oral and Maxillofacial Surgeons position paper on bisphosphonate-related osteonecrosis of the jaws—2009 update. *J Oral Maxillofac Surg.* 2009;67(5 Suppl):2-12.

326. Cartsos VM, Zhu S, Zavras AI. Bisphosphonate use and the risk of adverse jaw outcomes: a medical claims study of 714,217 people. *J Am Dent Assoc.* 2008;139(1):23-30.

327. Khan AA, Sandor GK, Dore E, et al. Canadian consensus practice guidelines for bisphosphonate associated osteonecrosis of the jaw. *J Rheumatol.* 2008;35(7):1391-1397.

328. Healey JH, Tyler WK. The role of orthopaedic surgery in the palliative care of patients with cancer. In: Hanks G, Cherny NI, Christakis NA, Fallon M, Portenoy RK, eds. *Oxford Textbook of Palliative Medicine.* 4th ed. New York, NY: Oxford University Press; 2010:558-572.

329. Saad F, Eastham J. Zoledronic acid improves clinical outcomes when administered before onset of bone pain in patients with prostate cancer. *Urology.* 2010;76(5):1175-1181.

330. Trotter CC, Pfister AK, Whited BA, Goldberg TH, Artz SA. A controversy: linking atypical femoral fractures to bisphosphonate therapy. *W V Med J.* 2011;107(2):8-13.

331. Sellmeyer DE. Atypical fractures as a potential complication of long-term bisphosphonate therapy. *JAMA.* 2010;304(13):1480-1484.

332. Puhaindran ME, Farooki A, Steensma MR, Hameed M, Healey JH, Boland PJ. Atypical subtrochanteric femoral fractures in patients with skeletal malignant involvement treated with intravenous bisphosphonates. *J Bone Joint Surg Am.* 2011;93(13):1235-1242.

333. Fizazi K, Carducci M, Smith M, et al. Denosumab versus zoledronic acid for treatment of bone metastases in men with castration-resistant prostate cancer: a randomized, double-blind study. *Lancet.* 2011;377(9768):813-822.

334. Smith MR, Saad F, Coleman R, et al. Denosumab and bone-metastatsis-free survival in men with castration-resistant prostate cancer: results of phase 3, randomized, placebo-controlled trial. *Lancet.* 2012;379(9810):39-46.

335. Anselmetti GC, Manca A, Chiara G, et al. Painful pathologic fracture of the humerus: percutaneous osteoplasty with bone marrow nails under hybrid computed tomography and fluoroscopic guidance. *J Vasc Interv Radiol.* 2011;22(7):1031-1034.

336. Trumm CG, Rubenbauer B, Piltz S, Reiser MF, Hoffmann RT. Screw placement and osteoplasty under computed tomographic-fluoroscopic guidance in a case of advanced metastatic destruction of the iliosacral joint. *Cardiovasc Intervent Radiol.* 2011;34 Suppl 2:S288-293.

337. McGirt MJ, Parker SL, Wolinsky JP, Witham TF, Bydon A, Gokaslan ZL. Vertebroplasty and kyphoplasty for the treatment of vertebral compression fractures: an evidenced-based review of the literature. *Spine J.* 2009;9(6):501-508.

338. Buchbinder R, Osborne RH, Ebeling PR, et al. A randomized trial of vertebroplasty for painful osteoporotic vertebral fractures. *N Engl J Med.* 2009;361(6):557-568.

339. Kallmes DF, Comstock BA, Heagerty PJ, et al. A randomized trial of vertebroplasty for osteoporotic spinal fractures. *N Engl J Med.* 2009;361(6):569-579.

340. Goz V, Koehler SM, Egorova NN, et al. Kyphoplasty and vertebroplasty: trends in use in ambulatory and inpatient settings. *Spine J.* 2011;11(8):737-744.

341. Gortzak Y, Lockwood GA, Mahendra A, et al. Prediction of pathologic fracture risk of the femur after combined modality treatment of soft tissue sarcoma of the thigh. *Cancer.* 2010;116(6):1553-1559.

342. Loblaw DA, Laperriere NJ, Mackillop WJ. A population-based study of malignant spinal cord compression in Ontario. *Clin Oncol (R Coll Radiol).* 2003;15(4):211-217.

343. Schiff D. Spinal cord compression. *Neurol Clin.* 2003;21(1):67-86, viii.

344. Sun H, Nemecek AN. Optimal management of malignant epidural spinal cord compression. *Hematol Oncol Clin North Am.* 2010;24(3):537-551.

345. Baines MJ. Spinal cord compression—a personal and palliative care perspective. *Clin Oncol.* 2002;14(2):135-138.

346. Husband DJ. Malignant spinal cord compression: prospective study of delays in referral and treatment. *BMJ.* 1998;317(7150):18-21.

347. Patchell RA, Tibbs PA, Regine WF, et al. Direct decompressive surgical resection in the treatment of spinal cord compression caused by metastatic cancer: a randomised trial. *Lancet.* 2005;366(9486):643-648.

348. Abrahm JL, Banffy MB, Harris MB. Spinal cord compression in patients with advanced metastatic cancer: "all I care about is walking and living my life." *JAMA.* 2008;299(8):937-946.

349. George R, Jeba J, Ramkumar G, Chacko AG, Tharyan P. Interventions for the treatment of metastatic extradural spinal cord compression in adults. *Cochrane Database Syst Rev.* 2015(9):CD006716.

350. Loblaw DA, Perry J, Chambers A, Laperriere NJ. Systematic review of the diagnosis and management of malignant extradural spinal cord compression: the Cancer Care Ontario Practice Guidelines Initiative's Neuro-Oncology Disease Site Group. *J Clin Oncol.* 2005;23(9):2028-2037.

351. Loblaw DA, Mitera G. The optimal dose fractionation schema for malignant extradural spinal cord compression. *J Support Oncol*. 2011;9(4):121-124.

352. Tancioni F, Navarria P, Pessina F, et al. Early surgical experience with minimally invasive percutaneous approach for patients with metastatic epidural spinal cord compression (MESCC) to poor prognoses. *Ann Surg Oncol*. 2012;19(1):294-300.

353. Dworkin RH, O'Connor AB, Backonja M, et al. Pharmacologic management of neuropathic pain: evidence-based recommendations. *Pain*. 2007;132(3):237-251.

354. Roque IFM, Martinez-Zapata MJ, Scott-Brown M, Alonso-Coello P. Radioisotopes for metastatic bone pain. *Cochrane Database Syst Rev*. 2011(7):CD003347.

355. Slattery DE, Pollack CV, Jr. Seizures as a cause of altered mental status. *Emerg Med Clin North Am*. 2010;28(3):517-534.

356. Grewal J, Grewal HK, Forman AD. Seizures and epilepsy in cancer: etiologies, evaluation, and management. *Curr Oncol Rep*. 2008;10(1):63-71.

357. Drappatz J, Schiff D, Kesari S, Norden AD, Wen PY. Medical management of brain tumor patients. *Neurol Clin*. 2007;25(4):1035-1071.

358. Mikkelsen T, Paleologos NA, Robinson PD, et al. The role of prophylactic anticonvulsants in the management of brain metastases: a systematic review and evidence-based clinical practice guideline. *J Neurooncol*. 2010;96(1):97-102.

359. Glantz MJ, Cole BF, Forsyth PA, et al. Practice parameter: anticonvulsant prophylaxis in patients with newly diagnosed brain tumors. Report of the Quality Standards Subcommittee of the American Academy of Neurology. *Neurology*. 2000;54(10):1886-1893.

360. Mirsattari SM, Gofton TE, Chong DJ. Misdiagnosis of epileptic seizures as manifestations of psychiatric illnesses. *Can J Neurol Sci*. 2011;38(3):487-493.

361. Devinsky O, Gazzola D, LaFrance WC, Jr. Differentiating between nonepileptic and epileptic seizures. *Nat Rev Neurol*. 2011;7(4):210-220.

362. Cocito L, Audenino D, Primavera A. Altered mental state and nonconvulsive status epilepticus in patients with cancer. *Arch Neurol*. 2001;58(8):1310.

363. Waterhouse EJ, DeLorenzo RJ. Status epilepticus in older patients: epidemiology and treatment options. *Drugs Aging*. 2001;18(2):133-142.

364. Lorenzl S, Mayer S, Feddersen B, Jox R, Noachtar S, Borasio GD. Nonconvulsive status epilepticus in palliative care patients. *J Pain Symptom Manage*. 2010;40(3):460-465.

365. Vecht CJ, van Breemen M. Optimizing therapy of seizures in patients with brain tumors. *Neurology*. 2006;67(12 Suppl 4):S10-13.

366. Swisher CB, Doreswamy M, Gingrich KJ, Vredenburgh JJ, Kolls BJ. Phenytoin, levetiracetam, and pregabalin in the acute management of refractory status epilepticus in patients with brain tumors. *Neurocrit Care*. 2011.

367. Lorenzl S, Mayer S, Noachtar S, Borasio GD. Nonconvulsive status epilepticus in terminally ill patients-a diagnostic and therapeutic challenge. *J Pain Symptom Manage*. 2008;36(2):200-205.

368. Miranda M, Kuester G, Rios L, Basaez E, Hazard S. Refractory nonconvulsive status epilepticus responsive to music as an add-on therapy: a second case. *Epilepsy Behav*. 2010;19(3):539-540.

369. Wudel LJ, Jr., Nesbitt JC. Superior vena cava syndrome. *Curr Treat Options Oncol*. 2001;2(1):77-91.

370. Rose D, Santo C, Frati G, Bizzarri F. Neoplastic superior vena cava obstruction: combined approach. *Eur Rev Med Pharmacol Sci*. 2011;15(5):577-579.

371. Lepper PM, Ott SR, Hoppe H, et al. Superior vena cava syndrome in thoracic malignancies. *Respir Care*. 2011;56(5):653-666.

372. Wilson LD, Detterbeck FC, Yahalom J. Clinical practice. Superior vena cava syndrome with malignant causes. *N Engl J Med.* 2007;356(18):1862-1869.

373. Gray BH, Olin JW, Graor RA, Young JR, Bartholomew JR, Ruschhaupt WF. Safety and efficacy of thrombolytic therapy for superior vena cava syndrome. *Chest.* 1991;99(1):54-59.

374. Greenberg S, Kosinski R, Daniels J. Treatment of superior vena cava thrombosis with recombinant tissue type plasminogen activator. *Chest.* 1991;99(5):1298-1301.

375. Halloul Z, Weber M, Ricke J, Smith B, Meyer F. Hybrid approach: vascular surgical and image-guided intervention for BroCa-induced superior vena cava syndrome (SVCS). *Thorac Cardiovasc Surg.* 2009;57(7):427-431.

376. Urruticoechea A, Mesia R, Dominguez J, et al. Treatment of malignant superior vena cava syndrome by endovascular stent insertion. Experience on 52 patients with lung cancer. *Lung Cancer.* 2004;43(2):209-214.

377. Duvnjak S, Andersen P. Endovascular treatment of superior vena cava syndrome. *Int Angiol.* 2011;30(5):458-461.

378. Kuppusamy S, Gillatt D. Managing patients with acute urinary retention. *Practitioner.* 2011;255(1739):21-23, 22-23.

379. McKinnon A, Higgins A, Lopez J, Chaboyer W. Predictors of acute urinary retention after transurethral resection of the prostate: a retrospective chart audit. *Urol Nurs.* 2011;31(4):207-212.

380. Sweeney A, Harrington A, Button D. Suprapubic catheters—a shared understanding, from the other side looking in. *J Wound Ostomy Continence Nurs.* 2007;34(4):418-424.

381. Lapitan MC, Buckley BS. Impact of palliative urinary diversion by percutaneous nephrostomy drainage and ureteral stenting among patients with advanced cervical cancer and obstructive uropathy: a prospective cohort. *J Obstet Gynaecol Res.* 2011;37(8):1061-1070.

382. Norman RW, Bailly G. Genitourinary problems in palliative medicine. In: Hanks G, Cherny NI, Christakis N, Fallon M, Portenoy RK, eds. *Oxford Textbook of Palliative Medicine.* 4th ed. New York, NY: Oxford University Press; 2010:983-995.

383. Hanks G, Cherny NI, Christakis N, Fallon M, Portenoy RK. *Oxford Textbook of Palliative Medicine.* 4th ed. New York, NY: Oxford University Press; 2010.

384. Foulkes M. Nursing management of common oncological emergencies. *Nurs Stand.* 2010;24(41):49-56.

385. Alifrangis C, Koizia L, Rozario A, et al. The experiences of cancer patients. *QJM.* 2011;104(12):1075-1081.

Index

fatigue (continued)
  definition of, 37–38
  etiology, 37–38
  management of, 38–42
  prevalence, 38
  reversible causes of, 39, 40t–41t
fecal impaction, 56–58
fentanyl citrate, 54t
financial problems
  anorexia-cachexia and, 32
  anxiety and, 10t
fluoxetine, 39, 42
forced expiratory volume (FEV$_1$), 5–6
fosphenytoin, 83
fractures, pathologic, 74t, 78–79
Functional Assessment Cancer Therapy, 1
furosemide, 16, 54t

gastrostomy tubes, 27
ghrelin for cachexia, 36
glycopyrrolate, 58
  for bowel obstruction, 59t
  forms of, 17
  subcutaneous delivery, 54t
  for thick secretions, 9t
granisetron dosage, 50t
guaifenesin for thick secretions, 9t

haloperidol
  for delirium, 67
  dosage, 49t, 68t
  efficacy, 70
  indications, 68t
  in malignant bowel obstruction, 59
  for nausea and vomiting, 46t
  subcutaneous delivery, 54t
hemoglobin levels, 9t
hemorrhages
  causes, 74t
  massive, 76
  symptoms, 74t
HIV/AIDS, dyspnea prevalence, 5t
homeostasis, acid-base, 6
humidity levels, dyspnea and, 11t

hydantoins, 83
hydration, artificial, 71
hydrobromide dosage, 51t
hydrocodone, rotation of, 13
hydrocortisone, 26t
hydromorphone
  for bowel obstruction, 59t
  rotation of, 13
  subcutaneous delivery, 54t
hydroxyzine dosage, 48t
hypercalcemia
  causes of, 74t, 77
  delirium and, 65t
  incidence, 77
  interventions, 77
  nausea and vomiting in, 46t
  surgical stabilization, 79
  symptomatic, 78t
  symptoms, 74t
hypercapnia, dyspnea and, 6
hypercapnic respiratory failure, 18
hyperglycemia, delirium and, 65t
hypernatremia, delirium and, 65t
hyperthyroidism, 31
hypoalbuminemia, 60, 77
hypodermoclysis, 27
hypoglycemia, 65t
hypogonadism, 31, 40t
hyponatremia, 46t, 65t
hypotension, cardiac tamponade and, 75
hypothalamic-pituitary axis, 38
hypoxia, 6, 66

impaction, nausea and vomiting in, 47f
incontinence, spinal cord compression and, 80
infections
  cardiac tamponade and, 75
  delirium and, 65t, 66
  fatigue and, 40t
inflammation, cachexia and, 30
intracranial pressure, increased, 46t
ipratropium, 9t, 65t
iron supplements, 57

sleep disorders, fatigue and, 41t

sleep hygiene, 38, 39

social isolation, delirium and, 65t

social problems, dyspnea and, 10t

somatostatin analogues, 59t

sorbitol for constipation, 57

speech-language pathologists, 24

spinal cord compression, 80–82

    causes, 74t, 80

    decompression, 81

    symptoms, 74t, 80

    treatment of, 80–81

spiritual advisors, 10t

starvation, cachexia and, 30

status epilepticus, 82

stress, eating and, 22t

stroke

    delirium and, 65t

    dysphagia and, 23t

    dyspnea prevalence, 5t

subcutaneous (SC) infusions, 13

superior vena cava (SCV) syndrome, 74t, 84–85

suppositories, 57

symptom assessment tools, 1–86

tamine mouthwash, 26t

taste disorders, 22t, 45

tension, eating and, 22t

terminal delirium, 70, 71t

testosterone for fatigue, 39, 42

tetracycline, 26t

thalidomide, 35

thoracentesis, 8

thrombocytopenia, 76

tracheostomy, obstructed, 9t

trazodone for dry mouth, 25t

tricyclic antidepressants, 57

tube feeding, 47f

tumors. see also cancer; metastatic disease

    bowel obstruction and, 56

    CNS, 46t–47t

uremia, cardiac tamponade and, 75

urinary retention

    causes, 74t

    delirium and, 66

    management of, 85–86

    symptoms, 74t

urinary tract infections, 65t

valacyclovir, 26t

valproate. see valproic acid

valproic acid

    delirium and, 65t

    dosage, 69t

    indications, 69t

    for status epilepticus, 83

vasopressin, aerosolized, 76

ventilatory support, 18–20

vertebroplasty, 79

vestibular diseases, 46t

viral infections, dysphagia and, 26t

vision impairment, delirium and, 64

vitamin B_{12} deficiency, 31

vitamin K, aerosolized, 76

volume overload, dyspnea and, 9t

vomiting. see also nausea and vomiting

    in cancer, 31

    reflex, 44

walking aids, 8

warfarin, contraindications, 76

wasting, inflammation and, 30

weight loss, 16, 34

Xa inhibitors, contraindications, 76

yoga, fatigue management and, 39

zinc for dysguesia, 31

zoledronate, 77, 79